Family Doctors Say Goodbye

Lucy M. Candib • William L. Miller
Editors

Family Doctors Say Goodbye

Shifting Grounds and Relationships

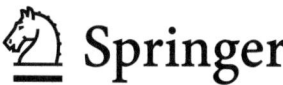

Editors
Lucy M. Candib
Family Medicine and Community Health
University of Massachusetts Chan
Medical School
Worcester, MA, USA

William L. Miller
Family Medicine
Lehigh Valley Health Network
Allentown, PA, USA

ISBN 978-3-031-33653-9   ISBN 978-3-031-33654-6 (eBook)
https://doi.org/10.1007/978-3-031-33654-6

© The Editor(s) (if applicable) and The Author(s), under exclusive license to Springer Nature Switzerland AG 2023
This work is subject to copyright. All rights are solely and exclusively licensed by the Publisher, whether the whole or part of the material is concerned, specifically the rights of translation, reprinting, reuse of illustrations, recitation, broadcasting, reproduction on microfilms or in any other physical way, and transmission or information storage and retrieval, electronic adaptation, computer software, or by similar or dissimilar methodology now known or hereafter developed.
The use of general descriptive names, registered names, trademarks, service marks, etc. in this publication does not imply, even in the absence of a specific statement, that such names are exempt from the relevant protective laws and regulations and therefore free for general use.
The publisher, the authors, and the editors are safe to assume that the advice and information in this book are believed to be true and accurate at the date of publication. Neither the publisher nor the authors or the editors give a warranty, expressed or implied, with respect to the material contained herein or for any errors or omissions that may have been made. The publisher remains neutral with regard to jurisdictional claims in published maps and institutional affiliations.

This Springer imprint is published by the registered company Springer Nature Switzerland AG
The registered company address is: Gewerbestrasse 11, 6330 Cham, Switzerland

To all our children and grandchildren and the younger generations who care about and advocate for the centrality of relationships, especially with our precious Earth and all its life and the overarching need to nurture and protect. Thank you!

Preface

This book is about the relationships we have with people in health care. Have you noticed the difficulty in finding someone, anyone, who really knows you? Someone who recognizes and appreciates your quirks, fears, special strengths, your hopes, some of your secrets, your story? This is especially true when seeking a family physician, a teacher for your children, a social worker, a nurse, or any other professional who recognizes the importance of caring, empathy, and relationship over time. Where have they gone? Many are retiring or leaving clinical practice and in greater numbers than those replacing them. The ground is shifting. Rooted in the historical traditions of the general practitioner, the Baby Boomer family physicians, the first generation of family doctors educated in three-year residency programs are retiring and saying goodbye to 40 50 year relationships with patients, colleagues, and others. And many second generation family doctors are changing roles and also saying goodbye. The disappearance of caring relationships triggered the development of this book. We have invited nine of our friends, leaders and pioneers during the first fifty years of family medicine's existence, to tell their stories, along with ours, about saying goodbye.

We share these stories to raise awareness of the importance of caring relationships when health is at risk. Saying goodbye is hard. The feelings of loss and grief are real, complicated, confusing like the relationships themselves. Caring relationships sustained over time are hard. They require commitment and even some sacrifice. And they are crucial nourishment for our health and our souls. Our world is rapidly shifting away from relationships to transactions in the false belief that algorithms, scripted customer service with a smile, and artificial intelligence will quench our deep thirst to be seen and heard. We profoundly disagree with this shift. The wonders and richness of life emerge when experiences are shared in caring relationships. We submit the stories in this book as our testimony.

We don't offer solutions or how-to advice but instead unveil the evidence within the stories that reveals the forces undermining healing relationships. Understanding and appreciating the problem precedes prescribing the fix. We believe in the power of stories to awaken the motivational energy for change. That is our purpose here.

We hope it contributes to a future where more people say, "Hello," to a healing relationship than are saying, "Goodbye."

We would like to send special thanks to the Springer publishing team that courageously accepted our book. In our personal lives, we are blessed to have an abundance of caring relationships with our families, friends, each other, our writing colleagues, and all the people we have worked with over the years in our practices and departments. We were especially blessed by the many thousands of patients who shared the wonderful and challenging parts of their lives with us. Through our time with all of you we have learned about the value of commitment and genuine caring. Thank you!

Worcester, MA, USA Lucy M. Candib
Allentown, PA, USA William L. Miller

Contents

1	**Changing Tides: Introductory Reflections** .... William L. Miller and Lucy M. Candib	1
2	**Cultivating a Goodbye to Harvest a Hello** .... Ann B. Reichsman	13
3	**Leaving Practice in the Era of Independence** .... John J. Frey III	23
4	**A Black Woman Department Chair Approaches Retirement** .... Jeannette South-Paul	35
5	**A Gathering of Crumbs, Stones, and Crows** .... William L. Miller	45
6	**A Stuttering Course to Retirement** .... Valerie J. Gilchrist	59
7	**For the Curious: A Brief Literature Review** .... Lucy M. Candib	67
8	**Facing Retirement: Grieving the Loss of Clinical Relationships** .... Lucy M. Candib and Eydie I. Kasendorf	79
9	**Retiring or Just Tiring?** .... Barry G. Saver	107
10	**Shy But Not Retiring** .... Kurt C. Stange	119
11	**When God Gives You a Good Kick in Your Rear End** .... Tochi Iroku-Malize	139

12	**Leaving My Patients, Losing Myself**...........................	147
	Cynthia G. Carmichael	
13	**Shifting Grounds and Relationships: Some Parting Thoughts**......	155
	Lucy M. Candib and William L. Miller	

Index... 159

Editors and Contributors

About the Editors

Lucy M. Candib, M.D. is Professor Emerita of Family and Community Medicine at the University of Massachusetts Chan Medical School. She practiced full spectrum family medicine with obstetrics for 40 years at Family Health Center of Worcester, a neighborhood health center serving low-income families including immigrants and refugees. After retiring from clinical care in 2016, Dr. Candib continued to precept residents and students until the COVID-19 pandemic. Working with medical students, she currently performs medical evaluations for persons seeking asylum in the U.S. Dr. Candib has lectured widely on topics of sexual abuse and violence against women and has drawn attention to the challenges facing women trainees. In her book, *Medicine and the Family: A Feminist Perspective*, Dr. Candib offered a feminist approach to family medicine theory and practice. Dr. Candib received a Fulbright scholarship in 1995 to teach family medicine in Ecuador. She received the World Five-Star Doctor Award in 2013 from Wonca, the World Organization of Family Doctors. Within Wonca, Dr. Candib has represented the Society of Teachers of Family Medicine, served as a member of the Organizational Equity Committee, and currently serves on the Executive Committee of the Working Party on Women and Family Medicine.

Family Medicine and Community Health, University of Massachusetts Chan Medical School, Worcester, MA, USA

William L. Miller, M.D., M.A. Lives unfold as stories and mine celebrates wonder, surprise, justice, and adventure. William L. Miller is a retired family physician, medical anthropologist, and Chair Emeritus at Lehigh Valley Health Network in the Lehigh River watershed of eastern Pennsylvania with more than three decades of collaborative mixed methods explorations of healing relationships, the general practice environments where they develop and how to improve them. Along with his friend, Ben Crabtree, he was awarded the Society of Teachers of Family Medicine 2014 Curtis Hames Research Award. Working with others, Will has co-created innovative research methods and educational programs, and founded a new academic community hospital-based department of family medicine with over 200 family physicians and their practices while also serving on national level committees and boards. His current work seeks to re-imagine general practice and primary medical care for the future and mentoring the next generation of family medicine leaders along with being an organizational rascal, occasional coyote, and grandfather.

Family Medicine, Lehigh Valley Health Network, Allentown, PA, USA

About the Contributors

Cynthia G. Carmichael, M.D. grew up in Miami, Florida. She earned her B.A. from Hampshire College and her M.D. from the University of California at San Francisco. She completed her family medicine residency in Miami, where she gained experience in the care of HIV+ patients. At that time, she and her brother, Kevin Carmichael, also a family practice resident, wrote an influential and well-received textbook, *HIV/Aids Primary Care Handbook*, together with an HIV specialist, on the primary care of patients with HIV infection. Their work led the way in integrating the care of the then highly stigmatized infection squarely within primary care. She went on to practice family medicine at community health centers in Richmond, California, and later at Kaiser Permanente for 8 years. During her career, Dr. Carmichael received multiple awards for her compassionate care, excellence in teaching, and superb outreach, including from such diverse organizations as the Dade County Health Education Center, the Jackson Memorial Hospital South Florida AIDS Network, the State of Florida Department of Corrections, the Contra Costa Regional Medical Center Family Medicine Residency Program, and from Kaiser Permanente the Teaching Award for Excellence in Clinical Medical Education.

Berkeley, CA, USA

John J. Frey III, M.D. is a descendant of Midwestern German farmers from Central Kansas, born in Kansas City and grew up outside of Milwaukee, Wisconsin. He was the first person from either side of his family to attend college, graduating from the University of Notre Dame, then medical school at Northwestern, and postgraduate education at Cook County Hospital and the University of Miami. He has practiced and taught family medicine since 1973 and since 1980 has been involved in faculty development programs, medical journalism and editing, and leadership roles in academic medicine. He enjoys encouraging faculty members to try new ideas, and it is a thrill to see when they successfully pull them off. The early stories of his life were usually punctuated with long Midwestern silences and understatement that taught him something about patience. His study of the lives of small town doctors has let him spend time visiting and listening to the personal histories of remarkable people. Since his retirement and becoming an emeritus professor, he has spent a great deal of time visiting with colleagues and talking about career trajectories. A friend who is a career coach calls himself a "whisperer" and that is how John thinks of much of his professional work these days. He spends a lot of time in coffee shops and over breakfast with people talking about career choices, personal growth, and strategies. He believes he is finally doing something that he thinks he is good at.

Department of Family Medicine and Community Health, University of Wisconsin, Madison, WI, USA

Valerie J. Gilchrist, M.D. received her M.D. degree from the University of Toronto, finished family medicine residencies in both Canada and the U.S., completed a faculty development fellowship at the University of North Carolina and the Executive Fellowship in Academic Medicine (ELAM). She is a past chair for three departments of family medicine—University of Wisconsin 2008–2020, Brody School of Medicine East Carolina University 2005–2007, and Northeastern Ohio Universities College of Medicine 1997–2005. She has received numerous awards and held leadership positions in most of the professional family medicine organizations. She currently is an Assistant Editor of *Family Medicine* and a Co-director for LEADS, a national mentoring program for those interested in becoming family medicine leaders. She enjoys health systems research, education, and patient care. After 45 years of patient care, she is retiring to write, travel, and enjoy friends and family.

Department of Family Medicine and Community Health, University of Wisconsin, Madison, WI, USA

Tochi Iroku-Malize, M.D., M.P.H., M.B.A. is the 2023 president of the American Academy of Family Physicians, past president of the New York State Academy of Family Physicians, and serves on numerous committees for specialty societies including the Society of Teachers of Family Medicine, the Association of Departments of Family Medicine, the North American Primary Care Research Group, and the World Organization of Family Doctors. Dr. Iroku-Malize is involved in diverse programs including, but not limited to, global and planetary health, clinical informatics, women's and children's health, special needs populations, cultural competency, advocacy, and leadership. She has worked for over three decades on clinical, research, and academic initiatives to enhance health and equity for both clinicians and patients across various communities locally, nationally, and internationally. A native New Yorker, she has lived in various countries and earned her medical degree from the University of Nigeria and did her internship in Trinidad & Tobago before returning to the U.S. She completed her family medicine residency at Southside Hospital and is dual board certified in family medicine and hospice and palliative medicine. In addition, she holds an MPH (majoring in health policy and management) from Columbia University and an MBA from the University of Massachusetts.

Family Medicine Service Line, Islip, NY, USA

Family Medicine, Donald and Barbara Zucker School of Medicine at Hofstra/Northwell, Hempstead, NY, USA

Family Medicine, Northwell Health, Hempstead, NY, USA

Health System Science, Feinstein Institutes for Medical Research, Hempstead, NY, USA

Eydie I. Kasendorf, Ph.D. is a licensed psychologist with 40 years of experience across a variety of clinical and academic settings. Her first contact with family medicine was as a psychology graduate student functioning as a scribe for the first Balint group in the new Family Medicine residency at the University of Massachusetts Medical School through the mentorship of her psychology professor (the Balint group leader). This experience led to her co-leadership of Family Medicine Resident Balint groups for over 26 years. In addition to clinical work that has included both community-based and private practices, she has also held teaching positions in the Clark University Psychology Department and UMass Chan Medical School Departments of Family Medicine and Psychiatry. These fulfilled her passion for teaching and supervising trainees across a range of health service professions. She also served on the Massachusetts Board of Psychology Licensure. Her professional activities illustrate her dual commitment to the needs of patients as well as to the professional development of other healthcare professionals.

Department of Family Medicine and Community Health, UMass Chan Medical School, Worcester, MA, USA

Ann B. Reichsman, M.D. is a dancer who wandered into the study of medicine when trying to balance her attraction to calculus with her love of humanities. She was immediately drawn to the new field of Family Medicine when she realized that this was where the rubber hit the road in implementing mind-body integration. After residency, a self-designed fellowship in Family Medicine and Family Therapy, and a 6 month research project in the Himalayas, she settled in Cleveland, one of the poorest cities in the United States, and joined a newly formed, nonprofit private practice in the inner city. She eventually became the Medical Director and then Chief Medical Officer of Neighborhood Family Practice (NFP) which grew into a Federally Qualified Health Center. In 1996 she was named the Family Physician of the Year for the state of Ohio and in 1996 was the Crain's Cleveland Business 2008 Health Care Hero, Physician Category. In 2004 she became the founding Chair of the Safety Net Providers Strategic Alliance Clinicians' Subcommittee, a practice-based research network in Cleveland. Since 2013, she has been a member of the North American Primary Care Research Group's Community Clinician's Advisory Group. She retired from active practice in 2022 and continues to provide informal guidance to her colleagues at NFP.

Neighborhood Family Practice, Cleveland Heights, OH, USA

Family Medicine, Case Western Reserve University School of Medicine, Cleveland Heights, OH, USA

Departments of Family Medicine at Lutheran Hospital and MetroHealth Medical Center, Cleveland Heights, OH, USA

Barry G. Saver, M.D., M.P.H. grew up in Aurora and Denver, Colorado. He then went to the northeast for college, graduate school in chemistry, and then medical school. He returned to California for family medicine residency, then worked in community settings in the Bay Area for 3 years. He moved up to Seattle for a 2-year research fellowship, getting an MPH and completing a preventive medicine residency. Over his 35+ year career, he engaged in primary care research, residency and medical student teaching, and clinical family medicine. He was principal investigator and co-investigator on a number of federal- and foundation-funded grants, with research interests focusing on access to care for vulnerable populations, organization and costs of care, and interventions to help patients collaborate with their clinicians to manage chronic health conditions. He stubbornly insisted on practicing in safety net settings, despite the limitations that choice sometimes placed on his academic job opportunities.

Swedish Cherry Hill Family Medicine Residency, Swedish Hospital, Seattle, WA, USA

Family Medicine, Emeritus, University of Washington, Seattle, WA, USA

Jeannette South-Paul, M.D. After medical school, Jeannette South-Paul, M.D., served as Medical Corps officer in the U.S. Army, retiring in 2001 while serving as Chair of Family Medicine and Vice President for Minority Affairs at the Uniformed Services University of the Health Sciences in Bethesda, MD. She then became the Andrew W. Mathieson UPMC Professor and Chair of the Department of Family Medicine at the University of Pittsburgh School of Medicine 2001–2020 retiring in 2020. In 2021 she joined Meharry Medical College as Senior Vice President and Chief Academic Officer becoming the academic leader of the schools of medicine, dentistry, graduate studies, and applied computational sciences. Dr. South-Paul served as President of the Society of Teachers of Family Medicine (STFM), and of the Uniformed Services Academy of Family Physicians (USAFP) as well as holding leadership positions in the Association of American Medical Colleges (AAMC), and the Association of Departments of Family Medicine (ADFM). She is a member of the Academy of Medicine of the National Academy of Sciences where she has served on committees evaluating Title X programs, veteran's mental health, primary care access for veterans' workshop, and the veterans' whole health program committee.

Meharry Medical College, Nashville, TN, USA

Kurt C. Stange, M.D., Ph.D. is a family and public health physician. At Case Western Reserve University, he is Director of the Center for Community Health Integration (CHI), which conducts collaborative *Research & Development for Community Health and Integrated, Personalized Care.* He is a Distinguished University Professor and Professor of Family Medicine & Community Health, Population & Quantitative Health Sciences, Oncology and Sociology. He served as founding editor for the *Annals of Family Medicine*. With Rebecca Etz, Ph.D., he serves as Co-Director for the Larry A. Green Center for Advancing Primary Health Care for the Public Good. At the Nova Institute he is a Scholar. With the OCHIN national nonprofit health information technology organization, he is an Affiliate Investigator. He is active in multi-method, participatory research and development that aims to understand and improve the generalist function, primary health care, health equity, and community and population health. He is a member of the Academy of Medicine of the National Academy of Sciences. Aware of the irony, he is stepping away this year from active clinical practice to make more time to try to bring to light what matters about a generalist approach to caring for individuals, families, and communities.

Center for Community Health Integration, Cleveland, OH, USA

Family Medicine and Community Health, Population and Quantitative Health Sciences, Oncology and Sociology, Case Western Reserve University, Cleveland, OH, USA

Chapter 1
Changing Tides: Introductory Reflections

William L. Miller and Lucy M. Candib

Background

A generational tide recedes as the next wave comes ashore. The baby boomer tide of family physicians represents the first generation to come of age at the founding of family practice as the twentieth medical specialty in the United States in 1969. They are also the first to complete 3-year family medicine residencies, and they are now saying goodbye to their clinical and leadership roles. Many saw themselves as participating in changing the face of health care to one that is more personal, relational, family- and community-oriented, and more equitable. They expected to shore up the foundations of primary health care, learning to care for infants, children, and adults, for the special needs of women, including delivering babies, and for overseeing patient care in hospitals, nursing homes, and emergency rooms. They emphasized a greater focus on health and integrating behavioral health and caring for the whole person in context. Many of the young women joining the residencies were highly sensitized to the need for women's health concerns to be directly addressed within family medicine and not in the more organ-focused and surgically oriented specialties. For 50 years, this generation of family physicians relentlessly pursued their vision. For the first decade, these hopes appeared attainable. But the last 40 years have been harsh to those dreams and efforts [1].

Recent commentaries raise alarms that, in both the United States and the United Kingdom, primary medical care, family medicine, and general practice risk an impending collapse as the overwhelming forces of neoliberal economics, global

---

W. L. Miller (✉)
Family Medicine, Lehigh Valley Health Network, Allentown, PA, USA

L. M. Candib
Family Medicine and Community Health, University of Massachusetts Chan Medical School, Worcester, MA, USA

© The Author(s), under exclusive license to Springer Nature Switzerland AG 2023
L. M. Candib, W. L. Miller (eds.), *Family Doctors Say Goodbye*,
https://doi.org/10.1007/978-3-031-33654-6_1

corporate capitalism, and commoditization fragment and corrode the health care system [2, 3]. The generational wave of family physicians born between 1946 and 1964 recedes from view and takes with them their embodied experiences of what's now at risk of being lost. As the tides change, what do they leave behind, what do they take away, and how does the tsunami-like incoming upsurge affect that? These are some of the questions addressed in this book. But there's more.

Sunset casts a glow over rooftops, western-facing walls, and billboards. A song drifts across the scene, heard by the housed and the homeless. Mourning dove, we suspect. One of those noticing the plaintive melody, Sage, sits alone in her upper-floor apartment. She feels ill. As twilight blankets the neighborhood, Sage seeks help from family and friends via phone, texting and social media, and she surfs the internet. But it's insufficient, and she's feeling worse. Where does she turn now? Darkness envelops Sage's neighborhood. With night comes the closing of physician offices. Her illness has a history that curls back in time through traumas and addictions. When Sage tries to reach out, who responds to her cry? Who says, "Hello, what troubles you the most?" Who sees her as a worthy person; who listens; who touches her suffering; who works with her to reweave her life and story back towards health? Will it be someone who knows Sage and has been with her before at troubling moments, or some well-meaning stranger on the clock following a protocol or algorithm? Over the last four to five decades, the family physician authors of the essays and memoirs in this book were there for Sage and for countless others like her, practicing their generalist, relationship-based craft of healing. And, as educators, they were often preparing future generations of such healers. Many were also there, working as leaders to facilitate the quality, organization, and delivery of this care. Now, they are leaving those roles.

Family medicine, along with many other service-oriented vocations such as education and social work, has passed through a turning point along the crossroads of history. For over 150 years (1850–2000), or nearly seven generations, primary medical care by physicians in the United States overwhelmingly consisted of small, usually solo, independent practices. The physicians were found in all health care settings, including patient homes. About 25 years ago, much changed. The majority of primary medical care practices are now larger corporate entities where care is segmented into billable elements, personal information becomes data, and increasing throughput (patients per session) is the primary objective. The majority of clinicians are now serving as employees in a retail market and not as independent professionals. Most of the changes named here had their origins in the 60s and 70s but didn't fully manifest until after 1980.

Nostalgia, especially that of white male elders, can blur our remembrances of the past. The historical general practitioners (GPs) of the early to mid-twentieth century in the U.S. are often fondly portrayed as pillars of the community where they had been embedded, always there and available. They often found themselves in a patient's home or their office in a corner of their own home, sitting or standing at the bedside of the patient with their stethoscope and black bag of remedies and injections. Norman Rockwell vividly painted some of these scenes; they still represent virtues and values that remain important. But, too often, we forget the shadow side of these traditional GPs. These include patriarchal paternalism, racism, a lack of transparency, an inability to assess quality, cures often worse than the disease, and high rates of addiction, suicide, and divorce among too many of those physicians. They had 1 year of training in hospital medicine and none in behavioral health. Meanwhile, post-World War II modern medicine made significant advances and, with that, began the rise of medical specialization. Fewer and fewer medical school graduates chose general practice. The briskly declining number of GPs available for a rapidly growing population reached a crisis point by the mid-60 s. Civil rights, feminism, Vietnam War protests and the counter-culture movement, environmentalism, and Great Society legislation related to the war on poverty, including Medicare, all swirled within the storms of this historical moment. Family practice, as the 20th specialty, emerged as one outcome in 1969, with 15 3-year residencies accredited at that same time. The concerns for justice, equity, inclusion, and environmental health nourished the roots of this new specialty. We hoped to preserve the virtues of the traditional GP, enhance and certify competency, and remedy the shadow side.

Family practice would rapidly grow during its first decade, with most of the authors in this book completing their residencies during that time. But alongside that growth came the increasing power of corporate mental models of practice, a consumer worldview, and innovations in information processing technology. All of these became more powerful forces with the election of Reagan in 1980 and went on to dominate developments in health care over the next four decades. The story has come full circle; family medicine, primary medical care, and all services dependent upon personal relationships over time are, again, at a crisis point [4]. Which brings us back to the reason for this book at this time.

As noted above, family medicine attained prominence by the 1980s. Now those early "adopters," the generation that began their careers as family medicine was being established, have done the craft for 30 or 40 years and are ready to leave it or transition within it. Some depart because of health or age, some in search of something new, and some out of frustration with the way the system no longer serves patients, disrespects relationships, and doesn't support clinicians. A second and third generation rise into leadership and administrative roles that reduce their clinical time and often involve a change of geographical location and displacement of relationships. Meanwhile, a fourth generation of family physicians and primary care clinicians is now answering the call as practice independence shifts to employment and information technology changes the interfaces of relationships. How do we speak across those different viewpoints and still honor covenantal relationships? The authors for this book represent pioneers and leaders within family medicine of major movements and changes involving issues of gender, race, research methods, power, training, and care strategies. They couldn't stop the tsunami of changes that has nearly drowned the generalist relational craft, but all participated, challenged, and lived with them. This book gives voice and grounding and some understanding to those sharing these experiences and to those now entering them. What happens when a family doctor or similar care-giving professional, deeply committed to long-term relationships, decides to end those commitments? How are they saying

"Goodbye"? This process of departing becomes, for them, a moment in time for reflection on what happened, what it meant, and what is already being lost. How are they imagining the future and relationships? What do they have to say to the upcoming generations about the value of relationships?

This book explores the questions from the point of view of the family doctors. Why the decision to leave? What's involved? What are the embodied experiences for doctor and patient, for doctor and staff, for physician leader, and others? What comes next? We invite you, the reader, to immerse in the personal stories and reflections of family physicians who choose to retire from practice, depart long-standing leadership roles, or shift from one place of deep relational commitments to something else. These stories concern the particulars of family medicine and general practice, but they share much with any vocation rooted in the duties, challenges, and rewards of relationships bound by covenant and not transaction and which are now at great risk.

What This Book Isn't

Since the pandemic of COVID-19, the media fills with news about moral distress, burnout, people leaving the healthcare workforce, and the accelerating retirement of baby boomers. This is not a book about retirement, although many of the authors have retired or are moving in that direction. We are among those leaving or changing roles. Many people are leaving clinical care to do something else, and yet there is almost no one talking or writing about anything besides "burnout" and what people need to do to take care of themselves as if it were just their lives that were affected, or they weren't resilient enough. What about a sense of calling? What happens to the many intensely meaningful relationships and to the others in those relationships? This book brings these questions to the center of the conversation. At least one and maybe two generations of physicians and other clinicians are pulling back from their clinical and leadership work now, especially since the COVID-19 pandemic, and many others are morally distressed because they can't maintain the relationships they have. They don't lack resilience; their agency has been stolen. All of you are the readers for this book, grounded in a relational standpoint.

It is not a book focused on reminiscing about the trajectory of a career in medicine and what has changed [5, 6], although some of that is present. This is not a book examining what to do after retiring from a life in medicine or how to manage the emotional aftershocks [7]. But careful reading will reveal some tips on these issues. It is not a book from the perspective of getting old [8] or on finding a new career [9], though some of the authors share insights on these topics. These are all important areas, and, as noted, there are already excellent books that spotlight these areas. This is not a "how to" book offering advice or guidance on retirement, changing jobs, or preparing for either. Rather, this book uses the power of stories and reflections to share the experiences of departures from cherished relationships and what follows. The authors' experiences are varied, but their need for change made them take the leap and then write about it, with relationships at the heart of that writing. That is what makes this book different.

Why Leave?

For the authors of the memoir essays in this book, deciding to change proved challenging and almost always involved a confluence of reasons. Ageing as getting older or turning 65 rarely factors in the decisions. True, you move a bit slower and need a couple of extra breaks or even a nap, but the brain remains sharp, and you embody decades of experiential wisdom. Unfortunately, the accelerating pace of changes in medical knowledge, technology, bureaucratic requirements and procedures, and corporate oversight make little or no compensation for those changes. Competence remains sound, but the constrictive context creates personal doubt. For several of our authors, the electronic medical record (EMR) system served as one of the last straws in tipping the decision point, in particular the EMR called EPIC. EPIC was designed by and works for a generation born after the mass deployment of screen-based information technology, and it was designed to maximize documentation for billing, not clinical, purposes. The computer savvy and agility required with typing, clicking, managing multiple screens, and intuiting the underlying "logic," and all for the wrong purpose, proved too morally distressing for some. But getting older isn't just about yourself. It also involves shifting family circumstances as the family life cycle turns: parents or a spouse requiring more support, and/or grandchildren needing help while their parents work. For two of our authors, serious personal illnesses further strained the situation.

Themes of abandonment, betrayal, vulnerability, uncertainty, identity, and fulfillment all surface in a complex mix. The relief of liberation from relational obligations combines with the grief over the loss of those same relationships and then merges with the guilt of letting people down. Regret and anger comingle with a heightened awakening of getting older. In many ways, the passages shared in this book officially acknowledge losses that have already occurred. These stories speak to all who have lost or are losing what was once sacred and precious to the current accelerating onslaught of change and commercialization. These stories both recognize the loss yet ultimately celebrate the abiding joy and wonder of relationships.

The Processes of Saying Goodbye

With the exception of the historical chapter and the literature review, the essays all represent a form of memoir. As such, we expect the authors to present their "better" faces to make their pasts worthwhile and meaningful. They are, after all, reflecting on choices made, surprises along the way, and, most significantly, the commitment of their adult lifetime to their vocation. How to self-appraise? How revealing to be? Do I admit to mistakes, and how many? How do I publicly reconcile the gaps between my highest aspirations and the more limited results? We don't have the whole story. Of course, we never have the whole story, including when performing clinical care. Nonetheless, many of our authors have been participants in Balint groups [10, 11] and are skilled at self-reflection. As such, they reveal much and offer many clues if you are willing to look for them. One of the keys to developing and sustaining effective relationships requires learning to peek behind the veil of others in respectful ways, sometimes leaving the explicit language unsaid to protect the sense of safety. Here are some hints on what to watch for and questions to ask about what you're reading.

Saying goodbye opens the often-guarded gate of wisdom; it begins to flow. Listen for it in all the essays as the river of wisdom flows widely in all of them. Notice the influences that appear to shape the experiences recorded. What experiences seem to matter? What troubles and problems surprised the authors by being helpful, especially when the writer learned to let go of control and be fully present in uncertainty? This skill of letting go becomes helpful when they must decide about saying goodbye. Again and again, you will witness lots of showing up and exploring, no matter how challenging or problematic the situation is. These authors, and all of those who serve others, have this amazing capacity for *being there*. Why? The authority of vocation and the call of curiosity keep surfacing as explanations. These folks love to learn, especially from others. Once there, they demonstrate well-developed staying muscles, even though most situations turn out differently than expected. Look at how they react, at their ability to recognize what's changed, and to adjust plans in mid-stride. They all recognize the importance of time and place. Observe it in their stories.

The hidden source of energy for these authors flows from the power of partnerships, from the relationships with patients to those with colleagues to those with family and friends. There are many stories of caring-in-relation and of sharing power [12]. Watch for this happening in all of the essays. This work of caring-in-relation generates an ongoing dance of distancing and boundary setting, protecting patients and ourselves while yearning to reach across for affirmation of friendship and competence. This dance represents part of identity creation, a process that's never complete and results in all of us being unique hybrids of multiple identities. Pay attention to this identity creation in many of the essays. This process serves as an important resource when the decision looms to retire or change roles.

None of the authors feel burned out from patient care; the EMR, bureaucratic hassles are another matter. The writers were there when patients needed them; they kept showing up for health crises and leadership challenges. They also have friends and families and creatively found ways to be present for them as well. And they all have lived full and adventurous lives. No, they aren't superhuman. No one is. But listen carefully to their stories, and you'll discover some secrets. The stories you read won't be about "work-life balance," since they all recognize that work is an integral part of life. They have all learned to compose a life, to piece together an aesthetic quilt of many patches woven from a moral fabric, a life of coherence despite the many irregularities and torn threads. The relationships supersede the importance of professional success. And yet, paradoxically, they have all achieved success. Listen for the trust, faith, and humility tucked behind their life choices, which help them maintain their integrity and their relationships. Notice the absence of the idea of legacy. It doesn't fit when relationships move to the forefront.

The stories reveal, both in content and in styles of storytelling, the reality and meaning of relationships in family medicine, in other such settings, and in living our lives. These shared revelations appear here at a time when they are being quickly forgotten or lost and offer younger generations a glimpse into the wonder and mystery of covenantal relationship and craft. The stories are so much more than nostalgia. On the surface, many of these stories of caring for patients or students or colleagues appear as "failures" and yet, how utterly powerful and healing they become. They help all of us re-imagine healing with deeper truth and understanding. They reveal the joy and the challenges of the art of relational care over time. The stories also highlight the importance of time and how to use surprise as a gift and not as a nemesis to be avoided. Health, for physicians and patients, often emerges from surprise. Welcome it in your own lives and work and watch for it in these stories.

None of the authors invited into this writing adventure are "really" retired. They've all made or are making significant passages out of leadership roles, out of ongoing continuity relationships with patients, out of full-time commitment to an employer and colleagues, and on to different relationships. They have all shifted into different ways of enacting their callings. The authors entered these departures for many singular reasons and are mostly still co-creating them. They are still composing their lives and piecing together their quilts. In our changing world, family physicians and others committed to continuity relationships move several times in their careers; they slip into and out of full- and part-time roles; they change employers; they undergo rapid and significant changes in how their care is organized and performed. They continue to move through the developmental life course and their family life cycles. How do they continue to honor the relationships that matter and manage these multiple changeovers? How do they honor their covenants? They see with their hearts. The storytellers in this book invite the readers to explore this question with them through their lived experiences.

Before entering the essay memoirs, we leave you with an older tale as a guide for your reading. Let us introduce you anew to the fable of *Br'er Rabbit in the Briar Patch*, first written down by Robert Roosevelt from the oral traditions of enslaved African-Americans and then made famous by Joel Chandler Harris in his *Uncle Remus* tales in the late nineteenth century [13]. These stories fell into disfavor when Disney animated them in their *Song of the South* with painful racist overtones. For our purposes, we wish to restore their radical, crafty origins. Br'er Rabbit represents a melding of African and Eastern Native American folk traditions. He goes back to Leuk, a rabbit trickster in Senegalese folklore. Leuk was converted to represent the Africans in bondage and became a folk hero to them. He was also blended with Nanabozho, the Great Hare from eastern Algonquian traditions. The story of the "tar baby" that we are sharing was borrowed by the indigenous enslaved people from a Cherokee folk tale. Br'er Rabbit is a trickster who succeeds with wits, not brawn, and provokes authority figures. Here's the story:

Br'er Fox (think dominant culture, corporate boss, plantation owner, etc.) is always thinking of some way to catch that rascal Br'er Rabbit and control him. One morning, he has a malicious idea and fashions a tar creature beside the road. Along comes Br'er Rabbit, who, always curious, looks at the tar figure and greets it. No answer. Now, here is Br'er Rabbit's great weakness, always looking for respect, not unlike family medicine and primary care. Br'er Rabbit gets offended and reaches at the tar critter to get its attention, only to be ensnared in the tar. Out pops Br'er Fox all excited. Br'er Rabbit begins naming all of the awful things that Br'er Fox could do to him and then says, "But, please, please, please, don't throw me in that awful briar patch." Which, of course, is what Br'er Fox immediately did. And off bounded Br'er Rabbit since the briar patch was his home. Br'er Rabbit remembered his purpose and place, the thorny briar patch of relationship-centeredness and undifferentiated sickness. This is where our authors meet their patients and colleagues, at these thorny edges of culture where tricksters live and healing happens along with equity. Relationships in the briar patch are where we thrive amidst a surrounding oppressive culture.

What's Coming?

The stories begin with the extended reflections of Ann Reichsman as she looks back over 40 years of practice and leadership in a community health center. We begin here because this memoir introduces several important recurrent themes. When the topic of healing relationships comes up, it's not unusual for most people to imagine an older, wise white male doctor and patients from a similar ethnic background. Neither Ann nor her patients fit that description. Many of the authors of the coming chapters conducted their clinical work in community health centers, where the patients represent the diversity of the human species and usually lack the material resources required by our profit-focused health care system. Seven of our 11 authors are women, and, more often than not, the author and their patients don't share the same ethnicity. Yet amazing relationships develop. Ann is a consummate clinician, and it is that work that feeds her soul so she can also lead her practice through turbulent change. These themes keep recurring in other chapters. She leads us through her process of changing roles and, ultimately, retiring, and how she cultivated her goodbyes in order to harvest a new life of hellos.

Now that you have a feel for what's coming, the next chapter shifts into a brief look back to before family medicine became a formal specialty. John Frey synthesizes hundreds of interviews and an extensive review of historical literature to help us appreciate retirement, or not, from a lifetime as an independent solo general practitioner (GP) before our current age of specialism, computers, and employment. For mainstream white medicine, this was the time of male doctors in private practice and segregated neighborhoods. Uncover the changes that profoundly shifted the grounds of relationships and the landscape of retirement.

Jeanette South-Paul brings us back to now and directly addresses America's original sin of racism and how it personally impacts doctoring, relationships, leadership, and decision-making. She transforms oppression into a vocation, one where retirement is not in the vocabulary. Until it is. Witness her creating change at the boundaries of power and now helping others do the same, a powerful way of saying goodbye.

The scene shifts in the next chapter to one where a privileged white male spends a vocational lifetime working to redistribute that privileged power and realign the healthcare system with its deeper purpose. He won't succeed on the big stage, but much is set in motion on the scale of human relationships. Will Miller also reminds us of how life constantly surprises us, disrupting plans and potentially opening us to discovery. He shares his journey through such changes as he also navigated the mazes of institutional culture and confronted moral distress. The EMR makes its entrance in this chapter. Throughout this process, Will gathers relationships to help find a way through.

Valerie Gilchrist brings feminism to the forefront in a personal and vulnerable way, giving it that much more power. A Canadian and a family doctor at heart, she reveals the challenges and surprises present in composing a life as a woman called to serve and how relationships shape and help with that process of composing. It's messy and not straightforward, with shifting family circumstances, self-questioning, and self-affirmation. It's filled with doubt and assurances, including the complicated issue of clinical competence. All of this is shared as Val slowly "stutters" her way towards retirement.

We pause, in the next chapter, to collectively catch our breath. Using a question-and-answer format, Lucy explores the literature on retirement in family medicine and medicine in general. She uncovers how little is written about relationships or even about the perspectives and feelings of the others, the patients, or the colleagues. She also describes the reluctance of physicians to reveal their emotional and more vulnerable sides, the places where caring-in-relation finds its source. On this, the literature is silent.

Until now. Lucy Candib and Eydie Kasendorf co-write the next chapter and open the door to the worlds of grief and loss. Lucy has spent her career seeking to restore power to those with whom she cares in relationship. She recognized how difficult it would be to say goodbye to 40 or more years of shared care and suffering and joy. She enlisted a psychology colleague with whom she shared a long-term interest in Balint groups to help her with the process of saying goodbye. The stories will challenge your expectations and assumptions. Relationships and "success" in caring prove to be richer, deeper, stronger, more fragile, challenging, and amazing than any idealized version. It gets real in this chapter. Take extra time to read.

Up until now, the authors all had extended periods of continuity relationships in their clinical settings with no or only two or three significant moves. Barry Saver moved many times. And yet, relationships still mattered and have been a saving grace through the multiple transitions. Barry is a master listener. This chapter explores how family, a powerful sense of purpose, and a sense of humor help him struggle through the changes and emerge, maybe more tired, but filled with gratitude and fulfillment in surprising ways.

All the authors of the preceding chapters have or are about to retire. That's not true for the next two. Kurt Stange writes about his sabbatical, a time out from the crazy-making in his life as a leading family medicine researcher, busy clinician, father and husband, administrator, and editor of the leading North American family medicine research journal. He describes the transformation that ensued and learning how to let go. Kurt takes us on his personal journey that results in his changing roles while staying in Cleveland, Ohio. Many relationships change, and some remain, but nearly all are different. Discover how it happened and how that helps Kurt re-define himself.

Tochi Iroku-Malize is also not retiring. She's currently the leader of the American Academy of Family Physicians. But it wasn't a smooth road to that place. Born in New York to parents from Nigeria, her journey required persistence, a strong sense of purpose, and many critical supporting relationships along the way. She shares all of this, but the need to say goodbye to some assumptions was triggered by a life-threatening illness that shook her foundations. They didn't collapse, but they shifted and transformed. Listen to the remarkable resolve and power of relationships.

Illness, in the form of Alzheimer's disease, serves as the antagonist in the next chapter by Cynthia Carmichael. This time, it does lead to retirement before it was desired. Cynthia, the family physician daughter of one of U.S. family medicine's founding fathers, Lynn Carmichael, describes the grief and loss, and love as her father slowly suffers and dies from Alzheimer's. And now, recognizing the early signs in herself, Cynthia uses words and poetry to courageously explore what it means to leave patients you love and to begin losing yourself.

The book concludes with some parting thoughts on the shifting grounds and relationships related to saying goodbye in family medicine. We welcome you to the shores of the heart where we have been responsible for those in our care. Enter our briar patches, with their uneven footing and prickly bushes, as we share how we are saying goodbye.

References

1. Miller WL. The story of general practice and primary medical care transformation in the United States since 1981. 2020. http://www.nap.edu/resource/25983/The%20Story%20of%20General%20Practice%20and%20Primary%20Medical%20Transformation%20in%20the%20United%20States%20Since%201981.pdf. Accessed 13 Feb 2023.
2. Miller WL. The impending collapse of primary care: when is someone going to notice? J Am Board Fam Med. 2022;35:1183–6. https://doi.org/10.3122/jabfm.2022.220145R2.
3. Abbasi K. Sunak fiddles while the NHS burns. BMJ. 2023;380:68. https://doi.org/10.1136/bmj.p68.
4. Hoff TJ. Searching for the family doctor: primary care on the brink. Baltimore: Johns Hopkins University Press; 2022.
5. Mizrahi T. From residency to retirement: physicians' careers over a professional lifetime. New Brunswick, NJ: Rutgers University Press; 2021.
6. Bolina P, editor. Becoming doctors: 25 years later: twenty five physicians sharing the journey from medical student to retirement. Franklin, TN: Clovercroft Publishing; 2021.

7. Romm S. Life beyond medicine: the joys and challenges of physician retirement. Hanover, NH: Dartmouth College Press; 2019.
8. Palmer P. On the brink of everything: grace, gravity, and getting old. Oakland, CA: Berrett-Koehler Publishers, Inc.; 2018.
9. Freedman M. Encore: finding work that matters in the second half of life. New York: Public Affairs, Perseus Books Group; 2007.
10. Balint M. The doctor, his patient, and the illness, vol. 234. London: Churchill Livingstone; 1957. p. 609.
11. Sternlieb JL. Demystifying Balint culture and its impact: an autoethnographic analysis. Int J Psychiatry Med. 2018;53(1–2):39–46. https://doi.org/10.1177/0091217417745290.
12. Candib LM. Medicine and the family: a feminist perspective. New York: Basic Books; 1995.
13. Harris JC. Uncle Remus: his songs and his sayings. New York: D. Appleton; 1880.

Chapter 2
Cultivating a Goodbye to Harvest a Hello

Ann B. Reichsman

Editors' Introduction

Mass media all too often misses the small local news that makes big differences in the lives of thousands of people every day and the individuals who make that possible. In Cleveland, Ohio, the national press failed to notice the color purple. For 40 years, a quiet, peaceful, and persistent force, a Family Physician usually dressed in purple, built, with her colleagues, one of the most successful federally qualified community health centers in the country, Neighborhood Family Practice (NFP). One of us (WLM) learned about this remarkable place of healing relationships while doing research on the role of complexity theory in primary care medical practices. NFP, as part of a local practice-based research network, had agreed to participate in a larger NIH-funded study. Within that study, a small number of practices were selected for more in-depth analysis. NFP was picked because it was clear from the data that something special was happening. It was and remains an exemplar that we fondly named Dusty Garden. One of the secrets was that Ann Reichsman was a lover of purple.

Ann's essay memoir aptly launches the stories in this book. When the idea of retiring finally enters Ann's consciousness, she activates memories from her earlier years, and the wisdom of decades begins to flow. Ann is first and foremost a clinician, and that is also what informs her leadership style and sense of purpose. She never wanders far from the clinical encounter and the relationship skills that were

---

A. B. Reichsman (✉)
Neighborhood Family Practice, Cleveland, OH, USA

Case Western Reserve University School of Medicine, Cleveland, OH, USA

Departments of Family Medicine at Lutheran Hospital and MetroHealth Medical Center, Cleveland, OH, USA
e-mail: areichsman@nfpmedcenter.org

honed in that setting. Read on and discover how it happened and how she says goodbye in a way that welcomes what's next.

Early in 2021, I realized that, in November, I would have spent 40 years working at Neighborhood Family Practice (NFP), a Federally Qualified Community Health Center in Cleveland, Ohio. In another month, I was going to turn 70. My equation became 40 + 70 = retirement! I had started getting the "When are you going to retire?" question about 5 years earlier, and my response was always, "I'm happy working now and I'll know when it is time." December 31, 2021, was clearly that moment as I was hungering for time without constraints and commitments, for days of waking up and deciding how to spend the rich, empty hours ahead of me.

Thinking of Beginnings

At the end of my career, I found myself thinking of the beginnings. The family that shaped me, the circumstances that set me on my career path, and the people whose guidance created inflection points along the way were all floating through my thoughts daily.

The path by which my family of origin came into being was wrapped up in World War II. My Jewish father was arrested by the Nazis in Vienna after the Anschluss and just before graduating from medical school. He was held in prison for several months and then, without explanation, released. After his last exams, he returned home to Yugoslavia and tried to impress on his parents the urgent need to leave Europe. He did succeed in persuading his father to send his sister to London for her education, and my father then set off for the United States for an internship. My grandparents, and his step-brothers, and their families stayed behind and most eventually died in Auschwitz. During his fellowship training, my Jewish father met my Catholic mother, who was at the hospital presenting her Master of Social Work thesis about the inadequate response of the welfare system to impoverished families. He was impressed by her and her work and by her warm greetings to everyone at this conference in Dallas, including the African-American attendees who were relegated by the hospital to a separate receiving line. He asked to be introduced to her. A courtship and marriage ensued despite her strong Catholic faith, which led to the children being raised in the Catholic church. I was the middle of five children and remember that one of our games was "Torturing Hitler." When I was 12, I discovered to my indignation that the Jewish faith didn't consider me Jewish but that Hitler would have killed me anyway. During my psychiatric rotation in medical school, I learned that it is unusual for Jews who experienced the Holocaust directly to marry outside the Jewish faith and that their offspring felt a need to make the world a better place. In my Family Therapy training, I read *Ethnicity and Family Therapy* [1] and was intrigued by Monica McGoldrick's description of conflicts that can occur in Jewish-Irish marriages. I recognized some of my family's dynamics. Examining my family influences made me curious about stories from my patients.

Most people are interested in talking about their lives, but there were those who found the process intrusive. When people felt comfortable enough to make a comment, I would explain my purpose and, when needed, pull back. Some went looking for a PCP (primary care physician) who didn't ask those kinds of questions. I might find out about a switch incidentally, most often when covering for a partner and finding a message that lets me know of the change. From there, it was a matter of conjecture as to what caused them to make a change. On the very rare occasion when I had a visit with a former patient, I would tell them that it was nice to see them again, leave an opening for an explanation if they wanted to comment, and I would compliment them on their choice of PCP. Since I often heard patients in various contexts feel that they weren't allowed to change PCPs, I wanted to put them at ease and make it clear that the power to choose is in their hands. If I felt miffed about the change, those were my feelings to handle. When I became the PCP for a patient switching from another clinician, I tried to remember to inform the former PCP. It sometimes became a teaching moment for a colleague and of course, their experience with the patient often gave me a head start on their care.

Dr. Hanna Faterson was a psychologist at my medical school with whom I had worked on a research project. I no longer recall what mistake I had made on my first home visit to a patient in the spring of my first year, but I'll always remember when I serendipitously encountered Dr. Faterson in the hallway right after I got back to school and said in a heartbroken manner, "I've just made a terrible mistake!" She laughed kindly and said, "And I'm sure that's the last one." That short sentence was immensely healing and was a lifelong influence on handling mistakes, leading me to collaborate with one of my colleagues, Heather Ways, on a presentation called "Medical Mistakes, Black Holes or New Galaxics," which suggested a procedure for handling the emotions triggered by mistakes and then gleaning the lessons from that mistake that would allow you to prevent the next one.

In my fourth year of medical school, I had the opportunity to do an elective with George Engel, the psychosomaticist who initiated the concept of biopsychosocial care. The elective taught me and the other student on the rotation about Engel's insights on effective interviewing, which shaped my work in a fundamental way. His technique involved eliciting a detailed picture of a patient's life at the time of the symptom onset, including their thoughts and feelings in addition to the standard medical questions, and then applying knowledge of physiology and human behavior to build the diagnoses. The careful listening, of course, produces its own benefits, both in the creation of relationships and the therapeutic effect of being heard.

When I graduated from medical school and started training at the Family Medicine residency at MetroHealth Medical Center in Cleveland, I was presented with disturbing surprises and challenges. The residency was grueling. Many of the eventual residency reforms had not been made yet, and unbeknownst to me, the Internal Medicine Residency at Metro was a pyramid program, which, even then, in 1977, was a relic from the past. During my entire first year, I was disturbed by an undercurrent of competitiveness when I rotated with the Internal Medicine Residents and then was shocked when suddenly some of the first-year group disappeared. I learned they had been cut from the program. It was one of those lightning bolt moments in which so much of the tension that I had experienced was explained. There would have been kinder ways for me to learn how much stress I could withstand, yet I did. In addition, I gradually became aware that I was uncomfortable talking to more than one person at a time. This presented a challenge when talking to groups of family members. Along the lines of "that which doesn't kill you makes you stronger," I found that the sleep deprivation, stress, and responsibility modified my introversion. The final touch in my journey to acquire communication skills came when Tom Mettee, the Residency Director, and I went to a recruitment fair. Without warning, he suggested that I go to the podium to make a speech about Metro Family Medicine. Although I was terrified, I agreed and managed to address the auditorium and apparently made enough sense to attract some candidates to our table. I graduated from the residency program with more self-confidence and the ability to make rapid decisions.

And that was good because my next step in training was a self-created fellowship in Family Medicine and Family Therapy at Metro. This involved attending duties on the inpatient service and working with Mario Tonti, DSW, our practice's Family Therapy Instructor. I saw families in a room with a one-way mirror and Mario behind the glass. We sometimes did co-therapy, seeing families together. It was challenging to act as a co-therapist with someone as accomplished and experienced as Mario. Although my tendency was to sit back and admire his work, his gentle and persistent pressure overcame my reticence. One of the earliest and most memorable sessions involved a couple in their 60s who had been arguing, for the entirety of their marriage, over an incident that had happened during their honeymoon. They had added more incidents over time that proved his thoughtlessness and her unreasonableness ever since. After the first and only conjoint session with them, Mario told me that some people just can't change; they are too stuck in their patterns. About 10 years later, I attended one of the Metro Family Medicine Grand Rounds in which Jack Medalie, the Chair of Case Western University's Department of Family Medicine and the initiator of the term "the hidden patient," was asked to interview a patient who was depressed. I realized that the person being interviewed was the wife of that couple. I was stunned to hear that, after our session, she and her husband had decided "that other doctor was right" and that they needed to move out of the past. They had a happy and fulfilling marriage until his death years later. This was an important lesson for me. We don't know what effect we have on our patients, what words stick with them, and how they might use our advice as they go forward with their lives.

During the stressful times in my residency, I used to tell anyone who would listen that I was going to leave right then and there and head off to Nepal! I wasn't kidding. I had seen a travel booklet about trekking in Nepal, and it called to me. So, when, in the Spring of 1981, towards the end of my fellowship, a physical anthropologist at Case Western Reserve University was looking for an MD to accompany her to Nepal, all fingers pointed to me. A few months later, I accepted a position as a National Health Service Corps (NHSC) volunteer at NFP, probably one of the last of that category before the Reagan administration closed down that aspect of the NHSC, retaining only the scholars. I was able to delay the start of that job until the fall, when I was to return from Nepal. My experience in Nepal was beautiful and deep, filled with new experiences, learning about the Tibetan Himalayan culture, and sharing exchanges with my anthropologic colleagues and our guides and translators. All of these brought new insights and a deeper appreciation of cultural differences. I was called to deliver a baby "that wouldn't come" the day that I arrived, and with that successful birth, I thought that many more opportunities would arise, but not until the day before we left did I assist in another birth. Apparently, the normal births were too routine to call for medical attendance. Fortunately, both complications were easily managed. In the first instance, it was a full bladder that was impeding the progress of the labor, and in the second, the same situation was preventing the delivery of the placenta. Working at a high altitude with just a few simple tools and the Merck Manual for guidance was a good preparation for working in an inner-city neighborhood in the United States and for the cultural differences that I would encounter.

It's All in the Neighborhood

After my return, I spent my entire post-training career working at NFP. I witnessed the opening of the practice, providing moral support to Barbara Toeppen-Sprigg, the founder. I refer to her when talking about NFP to prevent her founding role from being forgotten. Barb left after 5 years to pursue her long-held goal of specializing in Occupational Medicine, and I took over as Medical Director. Since I was around from the start, many people assumed that I was the founder. Barb had left me with a jewel of a practice, founded on feminist and humanist principles and focused on caring for the community as well as families and individual patients. I'm not a "founding" type person and not an administrative type either, so taking over as a director was not an easy process. I discovered that my training in Family Therapy was helpful. Systems Theory, which is so basic to Family Therapy, is also used to guide organizational behavior consultations, and there seemed to be adequate overlap to allow me to use what I had learned about systems to contribute to the management of a non-profit medical practice.

After Barb moved on to Occupational Health, the medical portion of the administrative tasks fell to me. I had 3 h every 2 weeks to handle the tasks that could be scheduled; the other ones were handled on the fly, either during patient care or after hours. Preventing burnout was a focus at NFP from the beginning. We were aware that many physicians start their careers in under-resourced areas but move on after a few years. We didn't want our people to follow that pattern. We had three (including me) part-time Family Physicians on staff, all of us mothers with young children. My work schedule when Barb left was two and a half days a week and gradually increased to three and a half over my 30 years in administration. A pattern of flexible schedules persists, and the majority of our clinical staff, including physicians, nurse practitioners, and therapists, are part-time due to their roles as parents or their life interests. As Medical Director and then Chief Medical Officer, I helped to keep NFP afloat through some really hard times, with a lot of the heavy lifting being done

Fig. 2.1 Ann and Sharon in exam room

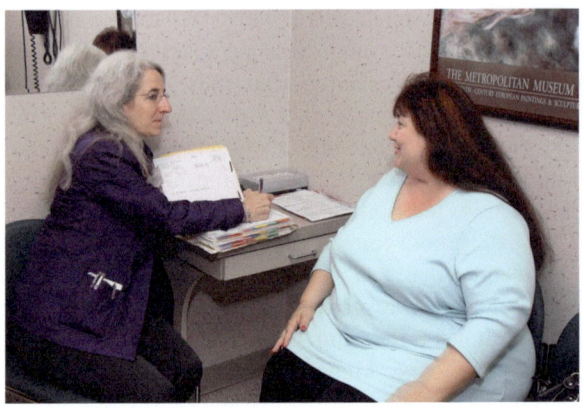

by NFP's successive Executive Director and then CEO as we became a larger organization. NFP grew in staff size and added new facilities, each nestled in its own neighborhood. My entire time as an administrator at NFP was only possible because my husband, Bruce Catalano, is a true partner. We both worked part-time and took equal roles with children and chores, except when he took on more of the burden at times when I became overwhelmed. When he saw that taking over a task would improve my life, he would add it to his load, and he never seemed to give it back to me.

In 2013, the size and complexity of the practice became more than my cobbled-together administrative skills and my energy could handle. I decided that I was interested in moving my efforts out of administration and back into the exam room (see Fig. 2.1). That change improved my stress level and allowed me to keep working for an additional 8 years. It raised some anxieties in my patients, as some of them thought that I was retiring rather than stepping back into clinical care. That gave me a preview of the disruption that the inevitable retirement would bring to the lives of people for whom I have cared.

Changing my role at NFP went smoothly. The challenges were to continue to be helpful while not meddling in administrative matters, to be available as a sounding board, to share lessons learned from our history, and to remind staff of our core values without undermining my successor. My ability to restrain myself was helped along by our new CMO, Erick Kauffman, and his organizational skills and his ability to tackle issues effectively.

The Long Goodbye

In January 2021, I knew that retirement was approaching, and I had conversations with Erick and Jean Polster, the CEO. We made plans to start the long goodbye later in the year. In the spring, I had a visit with a patient of over 30 years who is quite healthy and usually sees me once a year. I felt that it was important to tell her that next year she would be seeing a new clinician, so I did. As I finished the note about the visit, I had an "uh-oh" moment. "I haven't told the staff yet"! I scrambled to make plans for the announcement with Jean and Erick and continued to share the news with some selected patients, one of whom was the mother of a staff member. Annie, the staff member, kept the news to herself, and, as the staff meeting approached, I started sharing the news with my teammates. Jan, Natalie, and Donna, the team RNs, took it hard. Donna had often said that she would retire after I did, and then she double-crossed me by retiring 6 months before I did, leaving some of the most vulnerable of my patients feeling doubly bereft.

In the months leading up to retirement, I had some experiences where I felt I knew exactly what to say to someone in a very spontaneous way. I was seeing a 32-year-old man who has bipolar 1 disorder with psychotic episodes dating back to his teen years. I've known him since he was very young, starting as a toddler or kindergartener, and his behavior was consistently "completely inappropriate," according to his long-term therapist. He has been on antipsychotic injections and a mood stabilizer with long-term success, but seeing him is like interacting with the most obnoxious 12-year-old that you have ever met. He enjoys finding fault with anything that could improve his life, but this time, I called him on it. When he was done having a great time finding all possible reasons why he could not possibly find a system that would work for remembering to take his meds once a day, I pointed out to him that he was addicted to arguing. I leaned back against the wall, slitted my eyes, and said in my best junkie voice, "Oh man, hit me up with that argument man; it feels sooo good, man." He loved it, we had a good laugh, and we were finally able to figure out a system for him to use.

The goodbyes really started in the summer and fall as the time left in the year for the next appointments dwindled. The summer brought lovely moments of shared memories with my patients, reminding me of babies delivered, family members cared for, and important moments in our relationships. As the months to my leaving grew shorter, the visits became more intense, and I ended each day feeling wrung out with emotions. Most of my patient visits involved tears and hugs. My heart ached with their feelings of loss and abandonment, which for so many were awakening feelings from the many losses they had suffered in the past. Fortunately, NFP had recruited three new clinicians and, as part of their orientation, had set up Schedule Sharing with established practitioners. I was able to introduce my people to a new clinician, and we tailored the visit to the situation. Some of the visits were an introduction and, with the patient's permission, having the potential new clinician take over the visit until I rejoined at the end. Other visits were conjoint with the new practitioner and me both contributing to the flow. Although there were still intense emotions in these visits, I could see the new bonds being formed. I made sure to include some private time at the end of the visit to confirm the patient's comfort with the transfer of care and for an uninhibited goodbye.

Saying goodbye to Sharon was notable. She and I have been through so much together. I met Sharon in the 1990s when she came in to establish care for hypertension, diabetes, asthma, and depression/anxiety. Her husband, Larry, became a patient a few years later, needing care for occupational injuries, COPD (chronic obstructive pulmonary disease), anger management, and depression. In late fall of 2010, Sharon started having a lot of respiratory issues and saw several of my partners over the next few months, as well as having quite a few ER visits with diagnoses of asthma exacerbation, acute sinusitis, Bell's palsy, and a hospitalization for pneumonia. She was continuing to have very distressing symptoms and had an appointment with me in February. She described continued symptoms of Bell's palsy and trouble swallowing, as well as being unable to breathe when she was laying down. After more ER visits, she had an appointment with me, continuing to be in great distress, and reported that in addition to the intermittent left eye droop which had led to the diagnosis of Bell's palsy, she now had drooping of her right eyelid. It wasn't until I saw her having to hold up her lower jaw so that she could continue speaking that I realized that she had myasthenia gravis (MG). A long and complicated hospitalization followed in a specialty hospital where I was not a part of the team. I felt remiss in not having reached a diagnosis sooner. She felt I had saved her life. Maybe both are true. Our goodbyes stretched over my last 4 months of working. Each visit was marked by her anxiety for the future, aggravated by the continuing difficulties in managing MG and a new auto-immune disorder. The Schedule Sharing visit had gone really well. Our visit had equal input between her new PCP and me, fluidly moving from one of us making suggestions to the other. Her new PCP also demonstrated that her approach to Sharon was aligned with mine. The final visit in December was focused on the auto-immune disorder and the possibility that it may have been precipitated by the bovine pericardial patch that she had received when the malignant thymoma causing her MG was removed. Sharon cried off and on through the visit, and our final goodbye was through shared tears.

The hardest goodbye did not follow the usual pattern. Donna had been coming to see me for most of the 40 years that I spent at NFP. She was a rough-and-ready motorcycle mama who had no patience and spent any time that she had to wait for her appointment walking the halls and cursing. She was not interested in changing any habits or behaviors and took medications when convenient. As we aged together, she added chronic diseases and more treatments that she might or might not take. She harangued me about being late and not making her illnesses go away, but in the later years of our relationship, she started to say, "You know you love me," or "I love you anyway," even if I wasn't fixing her. As she added dialysis and amputations to her ailments and faced many near-death experiences, she stayed tough and defiant. I had a last visit with her 2 weeks before my final day at work. She was angry about the amputations, the phantom limb pain, and the continually recurring necrosis that signaled that more flesh would be taken from her. Her rant about doctors not doing anything to help her included me this time. I gently, without blaming, pointed out to her that her actions and refusals to act had brought her to this place, the edge of the end of her life. She made the fatalistic comment, "It's built into my body, there is no way to change it." She was sad, resigned, and then gave her characteristic laugh and said proudly, "I'm stubborn, not stupid and the dialysis nurses love me, I'm ornery but lively!" We parted as friends, and she died 2 months later.

As the final goodbye approached, I decided to set up a private Facebook group called "Keeping in Touch," and I created a "Doc Annie" account to use for that purpose. Doc Annie was my NFP name in the early days. Barb called me Annie, and the receptionist, also Barb, couldn't bring herself to call me by my first name, and since there weren't many people who could pronounce Reichsman, I became Doc Annie. This group was an important way to keep my personal Facebook page of many years private while still being in communication. I offered membership to a carefully chosen group of patients who had demonstrated their capacity for limits and had expressed an interest in having a way to connect. I made it clear with the invitation to join and the written material on the group page that this was for social, not medical, contact only. We, the patients and I, have mostly posted photos taken at various holidays or events of general interest, and boundaries have been respected. Many of us posted photos of our Halloween costumes, and there have been lots of cute baby pictures. One person posted about their musical event, and that turned into a themed thread of photos of our group members playing instruments. This summer, when I went to the Georgia Aquarium, I took a video of jellyfish that was so soothing it could throw you into a trance, and that was shared to wide appreciation.

Saying "Hello"

December 31st was my last official working day. About a month earlier, my sister-in-law, Laura, contacted our family to arrange a surprise birthday party for her wife, my younger sister, Frieda. The party was to take place in New England on January 10th, not really the time of year that I like spending 2 days along Lake Erie and Lake Ontario to get to the rest of my family in Western Massachusetts and Vermont. But then I realized, hey, I'm retired, no cancelled patients to worry about. If we hit a storm, we hunker down in some roadside accommodations until it passes by! So, we decided to leave an adequate time for bad weather and take a 2 week vacation visiting all my siblings, leaving Cleveland on January 6th. The travel was smooth, we were able to get both of our daughters and their partners to join the celebration and the party was phenomenal! We observed pandemic safety by having guests test the day of the party and no germs were transmitted at the event although one family was unable to join due to a positive test. Laura's birthday is 13 days before Frieda's. Laura had wanted to do a Beatles themed party for Frieda's 64th birthday in 2021 but was unable to do so because of the pandemic. Laura, who is an exquisitely talented hostess, told Frieda that she wanted to arrange a dinner party for her own birthday, but the invitees knew that the guest of honor was really Frieda. On the day of Laura's birthday, Frieda would still be 64, so the "When I'm 64" theme could go on. Laura collected all the needed decorations and accessories secretly and happened to crave for her birthday a dish that could only be gotten from a restaurant 45 min away from their home, giving us time to create the 1970s ambience complete with a life-size poster of the famous Abbey Road crosswalk (without the Beatles on it) for photo opportunities.

This serendipitous trip turned out to be the perfect introduction to retirement, framing my time going forward as an endless vacation. The reality, of course, is sprinkled with handling issues of aging and the expected obligations of caring for family and household, helping our house survive its own forms of decay, and taking actions that I hope will contribute to the survival and betterment of our species. Despite the challenges that we all face, I love retirement, the days that I craft for myself balancing exercise, reading, visiting friends, hanging out with my husband, and doing household chores. I have developed a new passion for replacing invasive plants with native species and got a persistent case of lateral epicondylitis by spending too much time pulling out English Ivy. We've traveled a lot, making up for some of the places we didn't go during the pandemic and connecting with far-flung friends. We even watched a full season of a TV show for the first time in a decade or two.

I'm grateful that NFP allowed me to have a rich career in the company of mission-driven coworkers at all levels of our organization and that the charitable community in Cleveland helped us overcome the obstacles to our growth and survival. I am especially grateful that so many people in our community opened their lives and families to me and allowed me to be a member of their stories.

Epilogue

When I made my plans to retire, I volunteered to help out if there was a need for a fill-in. Other retiring clinicians had done that, and as Chief Medical Officer, I had found it very helpful. After nine and a half months of waking up thinking, "What do I want to do today?" I got a call from Erick asking if I could fill in for someone on maternity leave. NFP was short-staffed, and patients were waiting weeks to get an appointment. I signed up for 2 half days, 8 h a week, which, with documentation and In Basket surveillance, gave me a 20-h work week. I made it through 3 months of fill-in. And I'm really happy to be done with that. I'm looking forward to returning to those unpressured days with my own expectations to guide my path.

Reference

1. McGoldrick M, Pearce JW, Giordano J. Ethnicity and family therapy. 1st ed. New York: The Guildford Press; 1982.

Chapter 3
Leaving Practice in the Era of Independence

John J. Frey III

Editors' Introduction

When questions about the history and philosophy of general practice and family medicine arise, John Frey's name quickly surfaces in the conversation. He has seen clinical practice throughout the different regions of the United States, worked with GP Julian Tudor Hart in Wales, been department chair at two prestigious universities, and served on the editorial teams of two leading family medicine journals. But friends of John appreciate him more for his travels around the country interviewing GPs and family docs, speaking passionately about justice and equity, worrying aloud about the future of relationships and community, and knowing the best local places to eat in so many small towns across America. Among his many interviewees were hundreds of GPs who began practice in the 1950s. In this essay, John synthesizes these conversations along with autobiographies to paint a picture of how GPs from this bygone time understood their relationships and thought of retirement. To be clear, he is mostly writing about medicine in "white" America, when most of our neighborhoods were segregated and white doctors saw few people of color, and those people often had no doctors at all. That has changed, but the inequities have not. That noted, the larger themes in this essay contrasting independent GPs with the employed FPs of today resonate with warning. The contrast with the current situation is dramatic, but the importance of relationships and community did not diminish with the next generation. The historical forces noted by John raise concerns about our next 50 years.

I have been interviewing family doctors over the past 35 years about their stories and professional lives and have read over a hundred autobiographies of general practitioners (GPs), mostly from the 1940s through 1960s. A lot of my

J. J. Frey III (✉)
Department of Family Medicine and Community Health, University of Wisconsin, Madison, WI, USA

colleagues have had parents who were also family doctors, and their stories have enriched my understanding of medicine in communities as well. Autobiographies are usually written for personal reasons. They sometimes don't contain much material on the struggle and failure that are part of everyday life. The stories I have gotten from my interviews and colleagues of mine with physician parents often fill in those gaps.

In 1968, a year before residency education in family medicine began, Fahs and Peterson published an article in *Public Health* [1] that predicted general practice and GPs would become extinct by the first decade of the twenty-first century. They may have been wrong, but they reflected the medical politics of the time in dismissing any potential turnaround as unlikely or impossible. They believed the gap would be filled by internists and pediatricians. Because GPs were retiring and saying goodbye, some reluctantly but many with a sense of relief, and there was no approved graduate training program, the future for general practice indeed looked grim.

Fortunately, by the 1970s, thousands of newly minted family doctors were showing up in family medicine residency programs around the country taught by hundreds of new faculty members. Many teachers in my residency training in the early 70s were either part-time teachers supervising residents from their private practices or were immigrants from long-time private practices who wanted to see a future for their communities and agreed, at great cost usually, to join or lead these new residency programs.

I remember hearing something about an older colleague contemplating "retirement," which was a word entirely foreign to me at that point in my career. I had signed up for a retirement plan offered by the university where I was employed but pretty much ignored it because I was busy doing my work of building things, not thinking about a distant endpoint. It would be almost two decades after residency training in family medicine began for the cohort of residency graduates to match the numbers of those leaving practice. GPs, who were now older family physicians, did not retire easily. They may have wanted to but were committed to getting replacements for their communities, and those replacements were slow to arrive.

Two major reasons that mid-twentieth-century general practitioners delayed or avoided retiring from their practices were concerns about sufficient financial resources to enable retirement and psychological issues about identity and meaningful work. Many had no plan for life beyond clinical practice. The first of those reasons, financial support, has, through tax changes, retirement plans developed by hospitals or large physician groups, and individually arranged retirement plans, become less worrisome and, in fact, retirement income for many physicians today is close to what they earned in practice. That was not the case at all when general practice physicians were less affluent in the mid- and even late twentieth century.

The second issue, the sense of purpose and meaning that practice gave physicians, continues to be an issue around retirement. Physicians who are committed to their practice partners have a sense of obligation to staff and to the community, along with a sense of responsibility to their patients. These responsibilities are tied up with the identity that family doctors have about their lives viewed as engagement in public service. That may be changing as physicians become employees, where the sense of ownership of the practice and oversight of staff is no longer present but rather determined by the health systems that employ them.

General Practice in the 1950s

For the greater part of the twentieth century, physicians functioned as small business owners "in private practice," a term rarely heard in the twenty-first century. Theirs were mostly individual or small group practices that offered an opportunity for buying into partnership. Physicians' families were often involved in the management of those offices, and payment was almost universally fee-for-service at the time of care and often with sliding scales responsive to individual patient financial resources. Insurance, which began to develop mid-century, primarily paid for hospital care and was slow to take hold until after World War II. Blue Cross, the hospital-based insurance, preceded Blue Shield, the physician insurance, by a decade. Until the era of practice consolidation began in the 1980s, primarily driven by financial issues like managed care and health maintenance organizations, physicians rarely considered a full retirement. Rather, they hoped for a scaling down of work and a lessening of the stresses on them and their families from the responsibilities of running an office. They longed for a time without the demands of the business of medicine and managing people. There was a well-known and successful U.S. Army recruitment advertisement that tried to induce doctors to leave practice by promising no paperwork or office management, just being a doctor.

During practice careers at this time, much of the advice given to younger doctors had to do with the cost-effective management of one's office. A great deal of latitude existed for physicians to charge or not and how much to charge or how to set up payment plans that met the financial situation of their patients. Taking time off for vacation was a personal financial loss. For long vacations, physicians often had to hire a locum tenens who was paid for session work. But new physicians, even those who joined an existing practice as a partner, were not handed full practices. Even if they bought an existing practice, the practice had to be built through trust, collegiality, and hard work. They were subject to up and down influences and, like any small business, suffered when there were hard economic times in their communities. They had to compete with other physicians in the community who were often less than helpful.

Guides for GP's starting practice in the mid-twentieth century focused on setting up a successful private practice. Stanley Truman, an active GP leader from California and president of the AAGP (American Academy of General Practice) in 1951–1952 wrote about the details of the beginning of practice, from choosing the community, the staff, the location, billing practices, and most importantly, in his mind, the relationship with other physicians in the community and region. Truman's checklist (see Table 3.1) [2] for physicians starting in practice emphasizes the relationships

Table 3.1 Checklist of what to do when starting practice in 1951

Select the community
Where do you want to live
With desired hospital facilities available to you
Select a location for practice
Parking, transportation, convenient druggists, laboratories, consultants
Select space, equipment, personnel
Arrange 24-hr. telephone service
Arrange with colleagues for emergency and vacation coverage
Get state license
Obtain narcotic license
Contact the county medical society and apply for membership
Call on doctors
Call on hospital manager
Become acquainted with the health department
Become acquainted with the coroner and his rules
Become acquainted with auxiliary health facilities
Contact insurance companies and apply for an examiner's appointment
Sign up for some charity service or clinic
Become a community entity
Join a church, synagogue, or mosque; join a service club; join a social or hobby group
Join the P.T.A or Dad's Club
Budget your time for:
Practice, community, medical organizations, home, and family
And live long and like it

Adapted from Truman [2]

between the GP and other physicians—specialists and generalists—and relationships with others in the community through volunteerism and joining.

Truman pointed out that the average GP's annual income in the late 1940s and early 1950s was $11,000. The photo essay, "A Country Doctor," in the September 1948 *LIFE* magazine stated that the average GP income was $14,000 while specialist income was four times that and more [3]. Truman wrote that the GP income was "sufficient … to keep the members of the medical profession free from want, in a state of security and responsibility and yet keep them out of the range where aspiration to wealth might become their ideal, …which is desirable from the point of view of the patient, the community, and the physician" ([1], p. 5). The irony of this statement is that the best solution for keeping physicians comfortable but not wealthy and also being the best for their community contrasts with twenty-first-century medicine. Today, employed family physicians often begin practice with $250,000 income guarantees and benefits to cover most professional expenses like malpractice insurance, and they require no investment in facilities and equipment and have no practice-based overhead. Tables 3.2 and 3.3 illustrate how much the times have changed.

Table 3.2 GP recruiting ads from 1950

Wanted: General practitioner for Utah County of 2000. Hospital being constructed within 30 miles. County adequately supported two doctors prior to war. No housing difficulty. Reply box A 112
For Sale: General practice that has been unopposed for 30 years. Office in ten room house arrangement. Coeducational college nearby. Practice is in Minnesota and doctor wishes to move to warmer climate. Reply to box A 114
For Sale: Well-established general practice and/or complete equipment and furnishings in excellent condition. Five room office in corner apartment house. Three to five year lease possible. Reasonable rental. Washington, DC. Reply box 10

Adapted from ads from GP, the magazine of the AAGP 1950

Table 3.3 FM recruiting email from 2022

Family medicine
• Employed position with $240 K salary and RVU bonus
• $25 K sign-on bonus
• Student loan repayment
• No hospital call required
• Full benefits package
• Area's largest non-profit, community-owned regional health system
• 475-bed hospital
• Largest full-service acute care medical center in the area
• Level II trauma designated ER
• Handle the highest level of trauma in the region
• Center of Excellence in breast imaging, cancer center, metabolic and bariatric surgery, and advanced stroke center
• J1 candidates are welcome to apply
One of the happiest cities in America
• Premiere destination for family or individuals
• Centrally located between New Orleans and Houston
• Excellent private and public schools
• Nationally renowned public university
• Forbes ranked the top city for job growth and opportunities
• Vibrant community and downtown area: Enjoy festivals, live jazz, blues and zydeco, sports entertainment, and incredible dining
• One of best food cities in USA—Rand McNally/USA TODAY best of the road rally
• Regional airport

Adapted from email to author

Truman didn't spend much time discussing retirement planning. What he did examine were the insurance types a GP should have—life insurance, health and liability insurance, and malpractice insurance. The latter was relatively new, and the universally litigious nature of healthcare had not gotten to the point of changing the practice and scope of practice. Truman devoted four pages to savings and investment, mostly to encourage physicians to have both and to ask a banker or accountant for advice ([2], p. 64).

Preparing for Retirement

Prior to Social Security, pensions, or retirement accounts, physicians had only the income from their practice and the potential liquidity from the sale of their practice to a younger physician to help them when they could no longer work full time. Like many in middle-class America, general practice physicians tried to find investments that would provide some financial comfort for them and their families once they left practice. Predictably, financial agents selling "sure thing" investments targeted physicians as likely buyers with some disposable income and some liquidity and who were likely to be able to get loans at local banks who saw them as solid financial risks. But cattle ranching, housing developments, and real estate ventures that promised long-term investment income often resulted in failed savings. Skills of running a medical office were rarely transferable to financial investments and decision making.

Some physicians left practice altogether and lived modest lives of retirement. Others found contract work. At one point, many of the directors of public health departments, correctional health, and some government contract work were retired general practice physicians, many without the training that would enable them to do that work confidently. A few were either recruited or sought administrative positions, such as chief of staff in hospitals in their community or region. Although not paying much compared to highly compensated hospital positions today, these part-time jobs helped physicians be better off than many other Americans. They could continue to work contractually after they sold or left their practices. A New York physician counseled making plans for leaving practice by bridging it with part-time work:

So, after a career of hard, stressful, and yet fascinating work, and as the result of careful planning for the future, the parable of Horatio Alger may apply. The physician can slacken his pace, change the direction of his work to make it more suited to his age and have time to enjoy life a bit more. In so doing he can continue to make a real contribution to medicine and to society and still end with his boots on but perhaps with boots of a different style [4].

Many of the articles and books written during the period of the 50s and 60s advised about investments, insurance, and other methods of saving and growing funds with an eye toward retirement [5]. Social Security provided a small, dependable income and was the first real opportunity for doctors to have a reliable source of income in retirement [6].

Beginning in the 1960s, physicians' Professional Limited Liability Corporations (LLCs) were allowed to be formed. They afforded some protection of the doctor's assets from malpractice suits but also allowed physicians, for the first time, to create and add tax-free revenue to retirement plans. At the same time, Medicare had gotten underway and served as an inflection point where medicine, as a good middle-class profession, became a source of real wealth for physicians. In the 60 years since Medicare and Medicaid began, doctors went from family trips in station wagons to sports vehicles, airline travel, and second homes. Money begins its pernicious erosion of the importance of relationships.

Working for the Man

Malpractice suits became more common in the 1960s, and judgments could be made which would wipe out a doctor's livelihood and savings. Malpractice insurance was a necessary nuisance in the 1950s, but 30 years later, it had grown to be one of the most expensive aspects of the practice overhead of GPs. Surgical and obstetrical components of practice were the highest costs as part of the formula for individual malpractice policies. Even when physicians arranged for group policies through their State Academy of Family Physicians or the State Medical Society, costs continued to rise. Malpractice costs were early drivers to decrease the scope of practice, with GPs choosing to stop assisting in surgery and widely deciding to stop delivering babies. Those two activities were among the highest income-generating aspects of general practice. In some cases, hospitals would support malpractice insurance costs to help retain physicians, but smaller community hospitals could not sustain the costs.

With the rise of large hospital systems, managed care, and restricted participation in insurance company networks in the 1980s, physicians started selling their practices for hefty prices. They left independence and became employed physicians of the system. Rather than sell one's practice to another physician, which, again, was the only liquidity that many mid-century GPs had and was the traditional process of retiring, GPs and FPs sold their practices, often for large amounts to insurance companies and hospitals. Because of rising debt, most new residency graduates couldn't afford these older practices. One of the benefits of employment was retirement plans to which physicians could contribute pretax income and to which employers could contribute. But realizing benefits from those plans often required a long-term commitment to a particular employer and could be modified, with difficulty, if the health system was purchased by another system. By the twenty-first century, this was frequently the case. Each system had its own benefits package, including retirement programs that were often incompatible with that of the previous employer.

Employment often meant trading professional autonomy, control, and personal choice about scope of practice for corporately determined compensation formulae and "benefits" based on the number of patients seen and documented charges. By the twenty-first century, physicians, hoping to leverage their hard work and practices for a more secure future for themselves and their families and patients, had become employees of large regional organizations built for maximizing profit. In the bargain, Mephistopheles won the cost of working for the Man.

The Effects of Retirement on Communities

The difficulties that GPs had with the financial issues around retirement may have played a role in the emergence of family medicine as a specialty and the creation of board certification. The campaign for the change from General Practice to Family Medicine came from a practicing community that saw few potential replacements willing to buy practices or move into solo or small groups, even as far back as the 1960s [7]. Physicians who were considering retirement realized the pipeline was empty and that the practices they had spent years building and maintaining would be left without physicians and their patients without care. The concern about physicians abandoning their community along with a continuing sense of responsibility for their patients drove many to pressure the American Academy of General Practice to support residency training in family medicine. They also used their political contacts to push state governments to demand that medical schools pay attention to the acute need of communities for family doctors.

Medical schools, for the most part, ignored family medicine and primary care or actively worked to undermine their roles in education and clinical care. Academic health centers misrepresented generalism as "without intellectual merit and too difficult to master" and supported deconstructed care—by "a panoply of competent functionaries" [8] as the editor of *The New England Journal of Medicine* put it. Community hospitals understood the growing threats to both their own and their community's future and were eager to replenish the supply of generalists by supporting residency education in family medicine. Disdainfully, academic physicians said, "most community hospitals have little to offer graduate medical education." They went on to note that "A few selected community hospitals have the potential to be teaching hospitals affiliated with medical schools" [9]. Despite this rhetoric, community hospitals provided resources and hired faculty members from their own budgets. They became a safe haven for generalist education to flourish, in spite of the dismissive attitudes of medical schools. In the twenty-first century, a majority of family medicine training programs still continue to be linked to community hospitals.

Family practices are important employers, particularly in smaller communities. They provide meaningful work for many—estimates are six to seven employees per physician—and affect community businesses from pharmacies to hospitals. People who travel to see their doctor also shop and do other things in the local community. One measure of the health of a small community is access to a primary care physician. Healthcare availability may be a point of decision for businesses whether to open branches or stores or factories in a community. Not replacing a retiring physician had, and continues to have, economic as well as health effects. This insight was especially noted by the independent GPs of the twentieth century.

Being Married to One's Practice

The emotional issues that GPs faced with retirement were equally compelling. While retirement age in the mid-century was primarily 60–65, many family doctors continued to work long past the time when they should have or even wanted to retire because they had an important emotional connection to their work.

None of us wants a physician who is not conscientious, responsible, or well read. The overwhelming emotion in many of the physician autobiographies from the mid-century is the positive feeling of service to patients and communities and the rewards that came from medical practice. But in talking with physicians about why they chose to retire when they did, two issues came up repeatedly, emotional and financial.

Practicing medicine was both an emotional strain and a financial one. This is not a new phenomenon, at least the emotional component. Physicians felt that as long as they had the mental ability to engage meaningfully with patients and the desire to be useful, there should be no constraints on their continuing to practice medicine. Of course, the aspects of clinical work that require hand skills and physical strength such as surgery, delivering babies, and some musculoskeletal medicine may have to be left behind. But the care of chronic illness and end-of-life care, well child and preventive procedures are all aspects of practice that could be maintained. There are many stories from communities about physicians who practiced almost until they died. Most notably, physicians with long connections with patients were inclined to stay until the end—either their patients' or their own.

Often, unfortunately, some physicians had not "kept up" and, for reasons of mental acuity, exhaustion, or physical fitness, continued to practice beyond the time they should have. Instead of stepping back from the stage, receiving the applause and recognition from whatever level that might come, and settling into something else, far too many generalist physicians looked into their post-medicine lives and saw nothing. They held on in desperation, not out of loyalty. States do have medical boards which identify behavior that is problematic, and remediation and assessment programs exist to help physicians who want some form of rehabilitation to do so [10]. But many didn't take advantage. In the end, physicians should be encouraged to consider the option of whether or not to retire. Physician "wellness" programs should be counselling physicians on how to make decisions to leave practice as well as how to remain meaningfully and creatively productive.

Unfortunately, the financial issues I mentioned earlier, rather than the love of medicine, were more often than not what kept physicians in practice. No one was coming along to buy their practice or assume responsibility for their patients or communities. The ones for whom it was easier to leave were those who brought their children into their practices—which was a surprisingly large percentage of doctors in the mid-century. While there could be pain in that arrangement, as sons and daughters found some flaws in their parent's practice style, on the whole, the transitions were often well planned and executed.

The National Health Service (NHS) in the United Kingdom understood the financial issues of retirement and replacement well when, from the outset in 1948, those who built general practices included an adequate retirement pension that enabled GPs to leave the field but also recognized that the NHS was responsible for their replacement, not them. That reality could be bittersweet in many situations, with newer, younger GPs less immersed in their communities than the senior ones they replaced. But the retirement structure in the NHS did not weigh GPs with the worry about abandoning a community that was often the motivator for U.S. family doctors to continue practicing longer than they and their families, and maybe even some of their patients, preferred.

Leaving Is Hard

The motivation and values behind those who enter medicine as a service profession and stay with it and grow as clinicians and people are what everyone in society wants in their doctors. GPs were, often, the most direct examples of those values and, in the best situations, help small communities feel safer and more vibrant. Young people today who choose family medicine as a career, for the most part, seem to share this same drive to better the conditions of their neighbors as physicians did in the mid-twentieth century. But today, lives and relationships are more complex, expectations are higher for an economically and physically comfortable life, and the opportunities that reside in a practice of one's own have become more difficult to achieve. Family physicians, too often, allow institutions and not-for-profit and for-profit corporations to choose where they will work, what their office will look like, who they will work with, what they must measure, and even how they should practice in exchange for a comfortable income and "benefits," the most important ones perhaps being loan repayment and retirement plans.

But older physicians I still know prepare for the stop date for their personal practice with a combination of dread and relief [11]. Like the NHS, corporate medicine in the US will take responsibility for replacement, even if that effort is longer and more arduous than in past years. Just like we cannot sell our houses to people who will treat our gardens like we have, it is often best to step away completely in these times. Similar to the mid-twentieth century, there are still opportunities for physicians to engage in part-time medical practice, but they often require travel and severe limits on what they can do.

Retired physicians of the past century often continued to live in the community they served for decades. Occasionally they moved away but their lives and families and social support were usually where they practiced. The etiquette of retired physicians was an important topic to cover. Mid-century physicians put their likes and dislikes and how they practiced into decades of ownership, not the financial as much as the emotional ownership of their own work. I remember driving around as a new family doctor in my first community, and the person driving pointing out houses and offices where the GPs that I was supposed to replace had worked. The pressure I felt was not from a lack of medical knowledge. I knew I either had learned or could learn that. But I wondered whether I would ever be seen in the eyes of the community as even a small replacement for the people who had guided them and their families as long as they could remember. Their physicians, whether deserving or not, were shrines to selfless service and loyalty to a neighborhood or community.

Most family physicians in the early and mid-twentieth century left something of value and purpose as they retired. They built offices that reflected their relationship with patients and communities. They built relationships as civic-minded members of their community, often initiating programs such as hospice, school health, and domestic violence shelters. They served in leadership roles in their hospitals. They were seen as people who made a difference in their communities. Leaving was hard but leaving without financial stability was almost impossible. That part of retirement is better today, but the shift from owner to employee has changed the relationships of physicians with their patients and with their communities as well. That shift is more than symbolic in that mid-twentieth-century family doctors created a level of trust between their offices and their communities. Today, that trust is mediated by corporate entities and employers. Personal medicine had deep components of satisfaction that may not be reproducible because of the organizational and economic structures of family medicine today.

References

1. Fahs IJ, Peterson OL. The decline of general practice. Public Health Rep. 1968;83(4):267–70.
2. Truman S. The doctor, his career, his business, his human relations, vol. 45. Baltimore: Williams & Wilkins; 1951. p. 258.
3. Smith WE. The country doctor: a photo essay. Life Mag. 1948;20:115–20.
4. Maynard EP Jr. Should we die with our boots on? Bull N Y Acad Med. 1971;47(11):1350–4.
5. Arkin J. A monthly check--panacea of retirement. GP. 1967;35(5):177–80.
6. Frost JS. Partial retirement with social security benefits. GP. 1968;38(4):181–4.
7. Pisacano NJ. General practice: a eulogy. GP. 1964;29:173–81.
8. Ingelfinger F. The physician's contribution to the health system. N Engl J Med. 1976;295(10):565–6.
9. Peterson OL, Bendixen HH. A critique of graduate medical education in community hospitals. J Med Educ. 1969;44(9):762–7.
10. Frey JJ 3rd. Forgiveness. Fam Med. 2001;33(10):779–80.
11. Loxterkamp D. When it's time to retire: notes from the afterlife. Ann Fam Med. 2018;16(2):171 4.

Chapter 4
A Black Woman Department Chair Approaches Retirement

Jeannette South-Paul

Editors' Introduction
Jeannette South-Paul is one of the first people I (LC) thought of writing a chapter in this book. She has a larger-than-life presence and has mentored many hundreds of trainees and faculty over the more than four decades of her career. As she describes it, she came up the hard way and overcame obstacle after obstacle to become the kind of family doctor who served her community, inspired medical students, counseled fellows and younger faculty, and challenged the medical and educational institutions that badly needed to change because they were trapped in old assumptions and rigid hierarchies. Now, stepping away from the role of department chair at an institution without a commitment to diversity and equity, she has taken on leadership at Meharry Medical College, where she will guide the multiple health education schools as they prepare trainees to face the ongoing challenges of racism and inequity in American medicine. She will no doubt continue her mentoring of those she has advised for years as well as attracting new mentees with her always fresh and enthusiastic welcome. Her generosity of spirit is a great gift to family medicine and to those of us fortunate enough to have worked with her personally. She attributes her accomplishments and persistence to her deep faith; what is clear to all who know her is that love for each person, for the community, and for our shared work in family medicine is the wellspring of her ongoing energy and the foundation of her life work.

When you are raised in the lowest economic quartile of the country but in the highest quartile for faith and service, the word retirement is not in your vocabulary. When you decide you want to be a physician at age 12 and direct every academic, community, and vocational effort toward qualifying for medical school, retirement is not in your vocabulary. When your heritage is from an island in the Caribbean where few go to college and no one in your family before you has earned a doctoral degree, let alone a medical degree, retirement is not in your vocabulary. When your parents labored running a rescue mission in inner-city Philadelphia for more than 30 years and you lived with them and watched them age while working 24/7 to meet the needs of the homeless and medically underserved of all races, ethnicities, genders and hues, retirement is not in your vocabulary. When you realize there are no well-heeled grandparents or benefactors to support your academic aspirations and you begin working part-time in high school through every week, long weekends, and holidays to generate the dollars to bridge your grants, scholarships, and unexpected needs, retirement is not in your vocabulary.

When you decide to join Army ROTC at an Ivy League university as the Vietnam War is winding down and where you dare not tell anyone you have chosen Uncle Sam and then accept an Army scholarship for medical school, retirement is not in your vocabulary. When you are accepted to several medical schools and choose the one where you struggle to get housing near the university and you have people demean you and those who look like you as they insist you will fit in if you rent this dirty unit but aren't welcomed in a better one, retirement is not in your vocabulary. When multiple counselors, teachers, bystanders, and discouraging advisors observe your melanin-infused skin and tell you that you are likely not good enough to join the elite who will excel in the medical profession, nevertheless you do. Retirement is not in your vocabulary.

So, for me, life has been a series of transitions and changes that I have learned to navigate by always having a goal on which to focus. My initial intention in applying for and accepting an Army scholarship for medical school was to serve the country to which my parents had so eagerly immigrated in the early 1950s, get the medical education of which I had dreamt for years, pay back my obligation, and then depart government service to work where my heart was in the urban, minority, medically underserved environment where I was raised. What I did not anticipate was the power of the relationships I would build over time and how those relationships would bind me to my work. Those relationships were anchored in people from across the globe, representing disparate faiths, political persuasions, and cultural beliefs.

They were the peers who welcomed me into their circles. When I arrived in Augusta, Georgia, I discovered I had nowhere to stay 1 week before my internship orientation was scheduled to begin. I was so excited finally to be able to have a monthly paycheck with benefits that I put earnest money down to buy my first house. I investigated the benefits and process for obtaining a VA loan, discussed it with my parents, and knew this option was for me. However, upon arriving in Georgia with my packed, brand new mint green Dodge Omni (of which I was so proud but which turned out to be a total lemon!) I discovered my unethical realtor had sold what I thought was my house to someone else. I had no idea what to do other than try to find an apartment that I could occupy immediately. A fellow intern, Craig Clark, whom I had met the year before when we were medical students rotating in Tacoma, Washington, was happy to see a familiar face, and so was I. He had coaxed me into climbing Mt. Rainier. "It's August, cutoffs and a t-shirt should be fine," he said. Until we ended up on a snowy prominence at 7000 ft, and I was an icicle. He began to take off one of his multiple layers—who knew!—to share his clothing with this urban Philly girl who had no idea what she would need. So, when I shared my frustration and homelessness with him a year later and in the first week of orientation, he directed me to his apartment complex and helped me secure an unfurnished, but thankfully unoccupied, apartment so I could start getting prepared to embrace my new career as an enthusiastic and well-rested intern. The carpeted floor and a few blankets were actually not too bad.

There were the patients who accepted me after initial reservations. I recall the white retired military couple who were initially assigned to my friend and fellow intern, Tom Anderson. When faced with this former Vietnam helicopter pilot turned family medicine resident as their assigned physician, they promptly refused to see this black South Carolinian! Tom expressed absolutely no concern, saying that after two tours in Nam and surviving, this encounter barely deserved mention! Our program director, with his quirky sense of humor, promptly assigned them to me. As I prepared to enter the exam room where they awaited their first visit with me, he pulled me aside and told me what he had done, smiled mischievously, and said, "Go get 'em and tell them you are their last chance to receive care in the best clinic in the hospital!" I promptly entered the exam room, introduced myself, and told them I had heard they refused care from a black physician, but I was willing to forget that and give them a chance to appreciate how well I could care for them. And... after they picked their jaws up off the floor, they agreed. We slowly but steadily forged a strong clinical relationship. How strong that relationship became was evident 2 years later when they heard I was getting married and asked me for a wedding photo. Although a little confused, I provided them with the 4x6 photo. To my surprise and delight, 6 weeks later they appeared in the clinic with a hand-carved clock on a stand with the photo and our wedding date embedded, something I treasure to this day!

There were those whom I mentored when they were in college or medical school and whom I wanted to see progress another step along their journeys… and whom I cheered when they got a new job, or an academic promotion, or got married, or had a child enter college. Each announcement warmed and embedded them deeper in my heart and reassured me that I had provided value to another. So many were no longer mentees but rather friends.

Then there were the mentors who affirmed that I was where I needed to be and the best one suited to address the latest challenge the Army faced. There was Mike Scotti, who interviewed me for my residency and then followed and supported me for decades thereafter, not only while he marched up the military ladder to become a general officer but also after he joined the leadership of the American Medical Association. And Larry Ehemann, who hired me for my first faculty position at the Uniformed Services University (USU); and Jay Fogarty, who became my incredibly supportive department chair and friend thereafter for many years. And Mary Dix, who helped me understand corporate and organizational culture in my first administrative position as VP for Minority Affairs; and Nancy Gary, who encouraged, educated, and sponsored me as a woman leader while she was the Dean at USU and for many years thereafter; and Val Hemming, who succeeded her as Dean and whom I told I was being invited to apply for a civilian position but knew I was unlikely to be chosen. He stopped me and said, "I would hate to lose you but am confident they will see how much value you could bring and will snatch you up!" After years of feeling I had to justify my skill and value as a family doc, having the support of academicians in Family Medicine and Nephrology and Pediatric Infectious Disease was unbelievably gratifying. I then felt I had a responsibility to embrace this journey and excel in reaching out and embracing others who might not have thought they had a place in the field of academic medicine and who could succeed and exceed the expectations of others!

Medicine can be any and all you want it to be, and it can offer more the longer you survive the medical career journey. I wanted to be a physician because my life from adolescence onwards highlighted to me the health and healthcare inequities of the community in which I lived. I listened to the struggles my parents experienced and how they needed to make decisions regarding whether they could afford to go to the emergency department for one ailment or injury for one of my five siblings and me—not to mention them—or rather use the few dollars for buying more food to feed their always hungry brood. I knew I wanted medicine to touch patients, to learn about their problems, and to help develop solutions. I felt privileged to learn about the most intimate issues impacting the well-being of my patients, but soon recognized that power comes from being able to influence the lives of larger groups and populations, especially the next generation.

When I was privileged to be selected as a department chair for the first time (while still in the Army), my plan was to stay as long as necessary to make a measurable difference. That meant expanding and developing the top clinical clerkship in the university, developing a faculty development program for remote adjunct faculty (at ten sites from coast to coast) and designing an annual clerkship teaching award, expanding our primary care sports medicine fellowship and adding a scholarly requirement, and developing medical student support groups for both women and minority students. It meant securing federal funding for a pre-matriculation program to entice minority undergraduates to seek careers in uniform and, subsequently, a postbaccalaureate program focusing on enlisted servicemembers who wanted to attend medical school.

When I retired from the Army upon being selected to chair a larger department in western Pennsylvania, I thought of the core goals for this position and committed myself to staying more than a few years in order to make a measurable difference. Becoming the first family medicine residency-trained family physician to chair the Department of Family Medicine for both the University of Pittsburgh and UPMC was itself a challenge. Then I discovered, upon beginning that journey, that I was the first woman and the first African American to chair a department in the medical school there, and I knew it would take more than a few years to make a measurable difference.

The complexities of managing and leading simultaneously in a region that had prioritized coal and steel, manly occupations, and corporate power and led the nation in those areas for decades were myriad. I soon recognized the importance of understanding my work environment, assessing the needs of those for whom I was responsible, identifying professional allies and concomitant adversaries, and establishing core supports to have the strength to manage it all. I also found myself surrounded by senior majority men who had been perfecting their craft literally for decades and showed no signs of departing. So I looked at every day as a test to accomplish something of value before I decided I had had enough and was ready to transition to something different. This is the story of my decision-making towards retirement, repurposing, reorganizing, and pursuing a quest for something different!

As I began my tenure as Chair of the department of family medicine in Pittsburgh, I knew I must prioritize key elements of my role since the responsibilities were substantially greater than I had faced while leading the family medicine department at the Uniformed Services University of the Health Sciences. I approached prioritizing my tasks similarly to how I had approached managing an inpatient clinical service. You saw everyone on service every day, determined whose conditions were critical, and then devoted the most time to the most seriously affected. I added one additional factor. My greatest attention would be directed towards the most socioeconomically disadvantaged because I did not see others with that same commitment. I recalled my experiences as a medical student, finding clinicians around me with little sympathy for patients of color, the less literate, the poorest, and those from the least prestigious communities. Indeed, the same populations who struggled when I was a medical student remained medically disadvantaged when I returned to Pittsburgh 22 years later; therefore, I finally wanted to make a difference. However, the overwhelming institutional priority, and thus a major focus for me as a department chair, was to operate in the black! No margin, no mission! Not only had this not been a priority while I was in the Army, it had never been an item for discussion. Rather the mission had been to care for those who cared selflessly for the nation!

I soon realized that this institutional priority blanketed literally everything we did in the department. I discovered the benefits of securing federal subsidies for caring for the poor, learned of Health and Human Services waivers through the 330 program, came to understand the pharmaceutical 340B discount program, found help in understanding the legislative acts that authorized federally qualified health centers (FQHCs), secured partners to help write the grant, and established the first FQHC at UPMC. I cut my teeth on negotiation by learning to partner with an outside discount pharmacy, mastered the tedious task of running an on-site drug dispensary, found a committed pediatric dental faculty member to staff our one dental chair to provide oral health services for children, and found skilled behavioral health professionals to care for the psychosocial needs of the population at our health center. The personnel, patients, laboratory, and administrative tasks were extensive but seemed acceptable when I saw how many uninsured, sometimes immigrant, and always grateful patients we were able to serve comprehensively over time.

I embraced the many pregnant women we served, but my heart ached for the teens whose lives were being shaped forever. So, I developed the *Maikuru Program,* named after the Shona language term from Zimbabwe meaning "big mama" or "wise woman of the village." We recruited teen mothers, partnered them with older women mentors (*Maikurus*), and met in small groups weekly, initially for 8 weeks for dinner and discussions and then later for only 5 weeks. The discussions were led by invited speakers to build skills to help them be more independent and successful as parents and successful citizens in a challenging environment. For more than 10 years, we were funded by local foundations to include the Heinz Endowments, who provided our initial, substantial funding, the Grable Foundation, who funded us several times, the Fine Foundation, the Poise Foundation, and the Birmingham Foundation, as well as support for our meals for several years by a committed leader at Giant Eagle Corporation. Our topics included contraception, spirituality and self-esteem, stress and depression, searching for and interviewing for a job, promoting education, and parenting.

The medical student education program was prioritized to include re-establishing a required Family Medicine third year clerkship. Dedicated faculty demonstrated their commitment to exposing our students to comprehensive, first-contact, coordinated, compassionate, and continuity-based care in the context of the family as a core commitment for the department. Not only did we dedicate a small group of educators to this course, but we also strongly participated in other courses such as medical interviewing, physical diagnosis, and electives such as cultural competence, family-centered maternity care, epidemiology, primary care sports medicine, global health, and primary care genetics.

What I did not anticipate when I returned to Pittsburgh in a leadership position after years of being affirmed as a leader in the military was that I was perceived as a token by many above me. My presence was to be an image for the community to serve as evidence that the health system embraced diversity. I saw myself as a lightning rod for expanding primary care to the wider Pittsburgh community, so they felt they had options for a personal medical home and training the next generation of family physicians. The system saw me as the black girl leading a department that would never make money. Family physicians were leaders in the military because it was widely known we were multidimensional and skilled not only as behavioralists and diagnosticians, but proceduralists as well. Whether in an ambulatory center, a classroom, the inpatient wards, or a combat zone, our colleagues wanted family docs. Many leaders were family docs and knew we were excellent anchors for any health enterprise.

However, this was not the case in a busy academic health center that had developed a 60+ percent health care market share in the region and bought every practice available to ensure their referral base. When I wanted to do the usual ambulatory procedures in our health center that were bread and butter in the military, we couldn't get support for the equipment and staffing necessary to provide the quality of care. Just refer them to the specialists. But the patients are more likely to adhere to our recommendations if we offer the services in their medical home. And we have the skills and the space. But no, that isn't why you are here. You are here to be a conduit of patients to those who really matter, the specialists, and can generate the largest profit margins for the enterprise.

Then hospitalists became the next best thing for reducing the length of stay and thus expanding profit margins. I knew family docs were ideal for this task as we were skilled in understanding the scope of care that was possible as an outpatient and thus could reduce the length of stay. In spite of developing a good proposal, they decided the intensivists should run some of the hospitalist teams and emergency medical docs the others. I couldn't help but wonder where the logic was here. Or was it me???

When I tried to interject discussions of community priorities in health system leadership meetings, I often found no one noticed my hand raised or my polite attempts to enter the conversation. I soon found two white male colleagues who were veterans of the enterprise piping in at times. "Let's let Jeannette speak as she has been trying to get a word in edgewise for a while!" they would exclaim. These trusted allies were important in keeping me in the game because these meetings often felt like a battle to reach the top! When it was announced we would spend millions on what was strictly a marketing move without an identifiable clinical return, I protested in the major morning meeting with all the clinical chairs and the CEO. I said the optics of this move will not be favorable to those we serve, especially those struggling the most. His response was, "That's why you are here." My interpretation being "to clean it up" for the public discourse.

As I became more vocal and less compliant, leaders were eager to tell me of opportunities outside the health system to get me out of their hair. I was approached for the newly vacated state health secretary position by the local state representative, who wanted someone from our region to run for this highly visible position. When I mentioned it to the school of medicine leadership, the response was, "Why don't you go to the state capitol to do that? There are opportunities in city government. Why don't you go do that?!"

When I received awards, there was little to no acknowledgement within the school. I was nourished by community recognition several times annually across numerous organizations while being ignored by my academic peers except when they wanted to recruit black and brown people in the community for research projects. The most significant event was probably when I was elected to the Institute of Medicine and felt absolutely ecstatic that there was finally recognition of years of commitment and value to the most vulnerable. Dozens of colleagues sent congratulatory emails. The Chancellor of the University, who has been an unfailing supporter, sent me the most gorgeous two-foot-tall bouquet of exotic flowers. My faculty held a surprise lunch for me at the University Club with a beautiful decorative gift. But there was silence from my immediate boss! Those elected the following year were feted, celebrated, and publicized in multiple settings over several weeks! I clearly recognized the message: you are still not good enough for our elite fraternity.

I soon realized that I had my personal and professional priorities, but my institution had its own priorities, and there was limited overlap. That is when I realized this position could only be satisfying for a time. When you learn the inner workings of an institution and more clearly see what is possible and what it takes to achieve each task, you realize the discordance in corporate versus personal mission, prompting you to engage in a decision analysis. What does personal success look like? You know how corporate success is measured, but how concordant are those goals with your personal goals? What are the additional goals you feel you can accomplish?

Who else can contribute to accomplishing these goals? How long will it take? What is your role in this vision—personal implementation, collaboration, mentorship, coaching, less or more?

As I worked through this process of analysis, I didn't believe those to whom I reported had moved much on issues of diversity. They recognized how my community engagement reflected well on the school of medicine and the health system, but they felt it was best implemented with money I could find elsewhere, specifically write a grant or convince a donor to support it. When I tried to reach out to the large local foundation whose recently deceased board chair had been a strong supporter of the university and after whom my endowed chair was named, I was told you are not allowed to approach them for funding. We are currently trying to get them to fund a major center at the children's hospital, and we don't want them distracted by your little ideas! I knew I had a vision for doing more, but clearly it was not the vision of the institutional leadership.

Yet I was gratified to recognize other younger faculty from a variety of disciplines who shared my passion for the medically underserved, were articulate about diversity and health inequities, who eagerly partnered with others to write and discuss these priorities, and embedded their passion in superb clinical care and institutional service. I realized there were others to whom I could pass the torch.

The other extremely important factor was rooted in my commitment to my family. For more than 10 years, I had been commuting back and forth 240 miles every other weekend since my husband was managing a busy surgical practice in the metro Washington, DC, area. Our sons and a nephew initially were in undergraduate and graduate school in Pittsburgh, so we were together and shared our love and passion for education in one location. As they dispersed across the nation pursuing military careers, and my husband and I realized that seemingly overnight we had become senior citizens with the associated challenges, the importance of facing those challenges, not only emotionally but also physically, together became a top priority.

When we pursue careers in medicine, especially those of us who are Boomers, we are ingrained with a strong sense of responsibility to our patients. This is not a responsibility to becoming skilled in electronic records or learning new technology, but rather in listening, touching, analyzing, and yes, embracing those who have entrusted their well-being to us! I struggled with considering leaving those with whom I had walked through pregnancies, returning to school, getting married, leaving traumatic relationships, managing chronic diseases, navigating complicated surgical procedures, surviving cancer, and surviving the deaths of children, parents, and spouses! Then patients must have begun to notice I was aging—more wrinkles, more gray hairs, walking more slowly. They started asking, no, telling me, "Don't even think of retiring! We cannot walk through these medical and life challenges without you." Initially, I felt affirmed and then challenged, but then I pivoted. My response began to be, "You know we have accomplished so much together, and I have hired some bright young docs who are actually smarter than me. You know you will never be left alone. If you stay here in this health center, these young docs and these wonderful, seasoned nurses, social workers, clinical pharmacists, and nutritionists who know you so well will still be here as your constant medical family, your medical home."

But although I had developed a narrative for my patients, the narrative coursing through my own mind was somewhat different. I had started this journey at age 12, defied the odds of growing up with poor, immigrant parents who were learning survival in the American economic system 1 day at a time, secured funding through one mechanism or another to complete my education, volunteered in many arenas to show my commitment to career, colleagues, and country, and worked 24/7. What would I do if I retired? Would I no longer be useful? Would I be remembered as having made an impact? But I would need to figure this out because I needed to make a transition while cognitively intact, energetic, and still brimming with ideas.

That is when I began planning my transition to leaving Pittsburgh and living again with my husband of more than 37 years. I envisioned sleeping more, exercising in the daylight outside and not just in a dark gym, traveling with my husband, and being with each other for our medical appointments and procedures. Several patients with whom I had journeyed for almost 20 years assured me that whenever I decided to leave, I would not lose them. They would write and call me to be certain I was taking care of myself. And they have!

So I chose a date, spent 2 weeks crafting a letter of resignation, and began my quest for repurposing. When I announced my decision in a faculty meeting, I did it through a slide presentation in the style of an annual report but covering 18 years. I reminded them of where we had started, what we had accomplished as a team, and why it was now time for me to move on. And I got choked up while saying the words. The word traveled quickly, and my dedicated health center team, i.e., my professional family, decided we should host a luncheon for my longstanding patients, especially the seniors, who would likely never have a clinical relationship with one person for so many years again. One young woman showed up at the health center at 0900, although the luncheon was scheduled for 1100. Our receptionist came back to my office and asked me to come out to see her because she needed to go to work and wanted a few minutes with me. When I walked to reception and saw her face, I couldn't help but smile. She had a bouquet of flowers in her hand, a gift bag, and a handwritten letter. She handed me the letter, and as I scanned the first few lines, I knew I couldn't read it then as I felt my eyes filling up. Then she grabbed me in a hug and told me how much she would miss me. "Do you know how you have raised me to be the woman I am today? I was 17 and pregnant when I met you and you promised to walk with me through my pregnancy, and then convinced me to finish high school and then the next pregnancy and then to seek further education so I could be a nursing assistant, and then showing me how to take care of my children, and always to keep moving forward!" She had recounted her memories of our relationship year by year for 15 years, even more than I remembered, and I knew I had made an impact!

In spite of the rivers of tears at the luncheon we held at the health center, and the gifts, and the heartfelt notes, and the hugs and more hugs and more hugs, I knew that transitioning from this part of my life was the right step. I could successfully move forward to the next phase of my life and continue to contribute to others without regrets!

What would I do next? The onset of the COVID-19 epidemic 2 months after I left Pittsburgh, then the death of George Floyd 2 months later and elevated visibility of the painful social justice inequities so pervasive in our communities, and the launch of medical student activism unlike anything previous resulted in my phone beginning to ring. Could we convince you to do a remote presentation for incoming first-year medical students on health inequities and racism at one medical school? Can you help our faculty understand what is happening in the post-George Floyd world from another medical school? And will you be a part of this advisory board for another organization, and more? Or calls from faculty from multiple schools requesting time to run certain experiences by me so they can plan a way forward. I realized I had not become obsolete the day I resigned and retired. Unlike the words of the Apostle Paul in the New Testament that I had always embraced, I have fought a good fight; I have finished the course; I have kept the faith. But I was not yet done! I had found a new purpose and more opportunities to choose my path!

What have I learned during these several decades in higher education, academic medicine, and life?

1. Be born into a supportive family that encourages you to dream! If you can't arrange that in advance, find surrogates such as aunts (genetically linked or adopted), teachers who love you and won't rest till you succeed, your own old-fashioned family doc because that is what drew many of us old-timers into Family Medicine, and/or mentors. Preferably, all of the above, since you can't have too many.
2. Develop a strong sense of self, an identity that is anchored in the knowledge that God placed you on this planet for a reason. Honor Him in your life and establish an integrity anchored in that belief that will allow you to be a servant leader who can withstand the ugliness in life that happens to you or is laid before you to handle in your day-to-day work. If you are not a leader, you are trailing behind and will always be covered in dust and swallowing what's left!
3. Cherish the family you have or the one you acquire so that they are with you at every step of your journey.
4. Surround yourself with generous and creative people of faith and integrity who will walk this journey with you and support you, and whom you support to create strong teams. Teams accomplish so much more than soloists.
5. Pay attention to your own health every day, no matter how noble the mission in which you are engaged. Pray daily, sleep soundly, eat right and in moderation, exercise daily, and love sincerely and for a lifetime.

Chapter 5
A Gathering of Crumbs, Stones, and Crows

William L. Miller

Editors' Introduction
I wanted Will to co-edit this book with me for exactly the aspects of himself that he describes in this essay: his commitment to a relationship-centered culture and innovative education. It had been clear to me from before my retirement that no one was addressing the various meanings that leaving a main part of one's career can hold. I wanted his big vision and larger-than-life presence to balance my tendency to get enmeshed in the details. When I first asked him, he was not yet ready to take on this new task, but over a 2-year period, the idea took hold. When expansion and prioritization of profit became the dominant values of the culture where he had championed compassion and innovation, he read the handwriting on the wall. He too had to go through the process of leaving what was not working and move on to new kinds of involvement while maintaining the deep and long-standing friendships with colleagues from his decades of relationship-centered teaching, practice, and yes, research. Collaboration in all these activities requires detailed attention to the relationships involved, yet no one was talking about what it meant to leave some of them and continue others in a new way. He began to say goodbye, first to patients and later to colleagues. He also had to say goodbye to a relational vision of family medicine, full of stories that he had invented and pioneered—Turtlecraft—in a Pennsylvania valley where his family had lived for nine generations and where he had taught decades of residents and young faculty. He readied himself to become a Tribal Elder. Sadly, he also became the Family Elder as both his parents died in the next few years. Yet he was able to integrate these losses in the face of the pandemic, when all were called upon to constrict their worlds and refocus on the close and the nearby. He both deepened his connections in the local community and broadened his family medicine

W. L. Miller (✉)
Family Medicine, Lehigh Valley Health Network, Allentown, PA, USA

© The Author(s), under exclusive license to Springer Nature Switzerland AG 2023
L. M. Candib, W. L. Miller (eds.), *Family Doctors Say Goodbye*,
https://doi.org/10.1007/978-3-031-33654-6_5

connections to collaborate in imagining a new kind of family medicine education for the future. His anthropology background reminds us that he will also be the one who tells the stories, preserves the culture of what has come before, and helps imagine with those coming up what might emerge afterwards.

Pappy's rocking chair came home from the office. As I hefted it towards the elevator, I noticed an observant crow perched on the ice hockey arena roof just below the eighth-floor office window in downtown Allentown. Twenty minutes later, the rocking chair arrived in our family room with a few crumbs on the seat cushion and a small Lehigh River pebble stone stuffed in my pocket. I settled into the chair, began rocking, and wondered, "Now what?" I'd left employment more than 3 years earlier but had preserved a small office space related to my Emeritus role. But now, with the COVID-19 pandemic and associated working from home, downsizing, and consolidating, my office space disappeared, and the rocking chair came home. Of course, none of this was part of the plan. Life and living rarely get the message about planning.

Becoming a family doctor wasn't even part of the plan. Neither was unearthing timeless love with my wife, adopting our daughter, returning to my childhood and ancestral home in the Lehigh Valley, discovering single malt scotch whiskey, or retiring from employment before 70. I'm an inveterate planner and an introvert, but to understand what happened in all these situations and so many more, you need to appreciate how I think about planning and relationships.

If change always happens to plans, why bother? I plan, in part, as a means for learning more about the landscape and its stories and for better preparing myself for those guaranteed unexpected surprises and changes. I also plan to gain more clarity about my intentions. Knowing surprise awaits around every bend in the journey, I like carrying significant objects from the past into the on-going present. Pappy, my dad's father, died in January 1960, when I was 10 years old. He was a quiet, enigmatic man, so unlike my father. He was the grandfather that I never really knew. I only remember him silently rocking in his dark walnut-stained mission-style rocking chair that may well have come from his childhood farm. When my Grammy died in December 1983, I requested that chair. I wanted it not only as a memory but as a daily reminder to learn more about those who sat in it. The rocking chair accompanied me through nearly 40 years of my professional life as an academic family physician and holds the memories of so many of the relationships that informed and sustained my vocation. Now it's come home. This memoir essay shares my experiences and perspectives on leaving employment as a family physician leader and teacher and on what happened to many important relationships.

This story unfolds in four parts. I begin with the decision to walk out of my role as Chair and walk on to something else, to reposition myself. That leads to the second part and co-creating, with friends and family, what renewal might entail. The possibilities filled the imagination with excitement, but the lived experience emerged differently. Thus, part three explores the maze of resetting purpose, relationships, and even time. Refreshment arrives in Part 4 as I rediscover presence in the moment and the relationships in front of me.

Part 1: Repositioning

The plan was to retire a few years after turning 70. I had been Chair since 1998. But somewhere amid 2015, I realized I needed to walk out of the Department of Family Medicine Chair role and walk into a different role as teacher-clinician-researcher with no further administrative duties. That's not what happened. I did walk out of being Chair in October 2016, but I also left employment only 3 months later, halfway to age 68. Everyone else called it "retirement." I named it "repositioning." Retiring, as a word, puzzles me. It seems to arise from the same mindset as "work-life" balance. When did work leave the realm of life? Retire derives from "to draw back into safety, seclusion." I left employment to change my vantage point, the position, from where I engaged the world. I did not seek to withdraw, find safety, or hide. I shifted my position to one outside employment, to one where the spaces for options and actions were more expansive. I was repositioning. But why not stay on as a teacher-clinician-researcher? What's going on here?

The change in plans had everything to do with relationships. My work in family medicine was built on relationships of many kinds. These included the obvious relationships with patients and practice colleagues and staff, but, given my multiple roles, they also encompassed relationships with the 120 additional practices in our department, relationships with colleagues in other departments, relationships with faculty and residents and medical students, relationships with senior management leaders, relationships with national and international research collaborators, relationships with the relational, generalist craft of family medicine, and relationships with family and friends. A brief detour into some backstory and context may help.

My wife, Deb, and I returned home to the Lehigh Valley in 1994, where I had the opportunity to start a new department of family medicine and a new residency in a place where my family had lived for nine generations, where my father had been a general practitioner, and where I had been in private practice for almost 4 years (1981–1984). I was beginning at the same time as a new Chief Executive Officer (CEO) for Lehigh Valley Hospital arrived with a vision for the health network to become the premier academic community hospital in America based on excellence, service, and innovation and with a local foundation willing to support innovation in family medicine education. Over the next 16 years, my colleagues and I co-created a relationship-centered culture and innovative residency and established ourselves among leaders in the field. Then, at the end of 2010, the board of the network replaced the CEO and did so again in 2014. The culture began to shift just as rapidly. It commenced with expansions, acquisitions, and an ascendence of a retail orientation and business focus. The shift accelerated with a weakening commitment to the local community and less innovation and more copying of others. A new idea in 2009 was welcomed with the questions, "How will it make us better?" and "How can we shape a business plan?" By 2015, new ideas were challenged with the questions, "How much does it cost?" and "Who else is doing that?" This shift was reinforced with a greater distancing between clinical leadership and the executive suite. Slowly but surely, the passion and commitment for innovative excellence and compassionate care throughout the organization eroded and made my own work and my many relationships much more challenging to sustain. The wheel of fortune had reversed direction.

By mid-2014, with the rise in moral distress related to these changes, I realized the need to make substantial changes, beginning with patient care. Little did I know that this was the beginning of saying goodbye. I was struggling to be there for my patients in any meaningful way. I was down to only half a day per week in the office and even starting to miss some of those precious times because of administrative distractions as our network expanded its geographic footprint. This expansion almost always involved adding more family physicians to our medical staff with many of them unfamiliar with our culture and expectations and often requiring frequent visits and even some retraining. My lack of availability to patients put added strain on my clinician partners and practice staff colleagues, and it wasn't honoring my covenant with my patients. I decided to stop caring for my own panel of patients and began what I thought would be the simple process of informing the practice and my patients.

Practice colleagues were immediately supportive and relieved. Informing my patients turned out to be quite another matter. I drafted a letter to send to patients and, in a spirit of transparency, shared it with the appropriate network department (marketing, of course), only to learn that they needed to approve it, and that my letter was not acceptable. I was duly chastised "to follow the standard retirement letter process" and given the customary letter to use (see Box 5.1). No way was that going to happen. I printed their letter and personally took the incriminating evidence to its source. I noted my offense at being referred to with the transactional word "provider" and that the impersonal and formal brevity were insulting to the more than 20-year relationships. "Sorry you feel that way; please just follow the policy," was the only response. I made a few minor changes to my original letter, sent the bureaucracy a copy, and then mailed it to my patients at the end of January 2015 (see Box 5.2). Officialdom responded with a reminder that it "shouldn't be insulting to anyone to use form letters," and, with a sense of exasperation, "…this mailing will be an exception." Patients were deeply appreciative. Over the next several months, I was able to see many of those patients for a "last" visit and, often, introduce them to their new personal clinician and hand over important stories.

I wasn't finished being an active physician. I kept my half-day in the office for another year but only saw patients with acute problems or those unable to be seen by their personal clinician. These were usually patients of resident physicians, and I discovered the joy of using these moments to both strengthen the relationship of the patient with the resident and to also suggest the next steps for the resident in the ongoing care of the patient.

In February 2015, the health network implemented the electronic medical record, EPIC, in all the primary medical care practices. For family medicine, this was the fourth different electronic medical record (EMR) since 1995 (Practice Partners, NextGen, and Centricity preceded). With each one, the difficulty of use grew more, and the clinical usefulness of the medical record became less. But, sigh, the billing improved, and the network could maintain a better watch over us. EPIC took all of this to a whole new level of trouble. I trained to become an EPIC superuser so I could help clinicians with their implementation. What I discovered was that EPIC and my brain were almost incompatible. Too many screens, clicks, documentation requirements, special keys, shortcuts, and checklists. The patient, their stories, my attentiveness, genograms, and time were lost to EPIC's voracious appetite. My ability to practice my craft of healing was compromised, and the moral distress was disheartening. I stopped seeing patients at the end of 2015. And I still miss it.

> **Box 5.1 Approved Provider Departure Letter**
> Date
> Dear_____,
> I am writing to let you know that I will be retiring as your physician effective _____. It's very difficult to walk away from years of providing care for so many wonderful people. But it's also an exciting time for me as I enter a new phase of my life and look forward to what the future might bring.
> I want to assure you that I am leaving you in excellent hands. Please contact the practice, and they will recommend another provider to continue your care. You can also get help in selecting another physician by calling _____ or by visiting _____.
> If you have any other questions, please call our office at the number on this page.
> Thank you so much for the privilege of serving you. _____ looks forward to working with you as partners in your healthcare for years to come.
> Sincerely,
> —

Here's the rub. I was a member of the network's senior management, chair of the department, and an early advocate for the EMR. Recognizing the potential value of EMRs but not paying sufficient attention to their consequences or how they were likely to be designed, I introduced the first EMR into the network and encouraged its spread. I still believe they could be redesigned to enhance the care of patients rather than billing, but it will take a complete revamping that is nowhere on the horizon. EPIC was a tipping point for me. EPIC arrived following several years of trying to hold back the culture of management changes flooding our network. Despite multiple efforts, I had not yet succeeded in getting our family physicians off the hamster wheel of a piecemeal fee for a documentation-based productivity compensation plan. This was made worse by the addition of pay-for-performance on specific disease-based metrics that ignored individual differences and capacities. It became painful and too hard to watch as colleagues struggled to meet productivity and performance expectations and use EPIC, something I could no longer do myself.

> **Box 5.2 The Retirement Letter Sent**
> January 31, 2015.
> Dear _____,
> Partnering with you as your family doctor on your journey of health has filled my life with joy, humility, inspiration, and gratitude. Thus, with many mixed emotions, I am writing to let you know of my intention to stop seeing my own patients as of July 1, 2015. As you are all too aware, for the past several years, my administrative, teaching, and research activities have made it increasingly difficult for me to have regular office hours. Thank you for your patience with my frequent lack of availability; I am sorry for that. Fortunately, you have also learned that our practice has some of the most knowledgeable and caring clinicians in the country, and I hope that you select one of them for your future healthcare. [Usually added a suggestion here.]
> I am not retiring. I am ending my regular practice so I can more intensely focus on other activities. I am remaining as Chair of the Department of Family Medicine and will also continue participating in resident and medical student education and in several national primary care research and policy initiatives. We are in a time of unprecedented change both in the world and in healthcare. As you probably know, I care passionately about ensuring that everyone in our community has the opportunity to be as healthy as possible. It is towards this goal that my energies will be directed. This will include working with and mentoring the primary care clinicians of our community as all of us seek to fulfill this dream.
> If you have questions, you can contact [name of person they know] at _____. She will also know how to reach me if necessary. [Information on the safety of medical records & how to transfer if desired.]
> What a remarkable privilege getting to meet and share in your care. I will deeply miss our times together and will always treasure the gift of our relationship. Your demonstrated strengths in difficult times were a source of inspiration and encouragement for my colleagues and me. Please remember what a remarkable person you are! I wish you continued good health and all the best in the coming years.
> Sincerely yours,
> [Usually added a personal note here, and I cried.]

I collided with my mirror of personal integrity, and the glass broke. My leadership style requires honesty, trust, transparency, role modeling, and relationships. These, in turn, require staying connected and knowing each other. With the health network planning even more expansions beyond the scale of my ability to develop and sustain relationships, the relational aspects of leadership no longer seemed possible for me. I needed to delegate them to others while I focused on senior management relationships and mentoring/coaching the younger leaders. Doable but not nearly as much fun, especially as the creative tension between business and profession succumbed to the sole dominance of the retail/consumer mindset. I peered into a smaller mirror. The glass held, but the view was unsettling.

Let's pause for a moment to reflect on what happened to the craft of family medicine and to those, like myself, practicing that craft. In earlier times (the 1970s and 1980s) of small, independent practices, we were able to align how we practiced the craft, how we assured competence, and how we maintained a clinical record. This alignment also included how we achieved our income goals, how we secured a good reputation with patients and colleagues, and how we safeguarded the quality and composition of our staff or team. We had a purpose, agency, and means for achieving mastery. The ability to weave these strands into a whole has since been disassembled and put into the hands of multiple managers focused on budgets and efficiency and brand. Stories shared between patient and physician look like a waste to these managers rather than the crucial food of relational health over time. Staff are hired and replaced by managers following human resource policies. Reputation is measured as patient satisfaction scores; income goals are achieved by producing more and achieving targets unrelated to excellent personalized care. The clinical record content is dictated by EMR requirements, and the ability to practice your craft at its best is nearly impossible. We lost agency; our purpose faded from the horizon, and the possibility of mastery was disappearing. Moral distress pervades. This was true for me, and it was what I was witnessing among too many of my colleagues, who were both friends and those whom I served as department Chair. Now what?

On January 4, 2016, I announced to all the Chairs, to senior leadership, and to the family medicine department that I would leave the Chair position in September (see Box 5.3). I felt new energy and joy as my work shifted to preparing the department, the network, my family, and myself for the transition, for succession planning, and for my own repositioning. It helped that I wasn't planning on moving or disappearing. I accelerated work on a five-year primary care strategic plan initiated 2 years earlier with leaders in general internal medicine and pediatrics (Note: that strategy is now far along in its implementation), and I intensified leadership mentoring of several of our younger faculty members and full-time clinicians (note: nearly all of them are currently in major leadership roles). My friend and truth-teller, Julie, who was the Department Vice-Chair and Residency Program Director, strengthened her mentoring of future residency leaders as well, since she was considering retiring shortly after me. This emphasis on succession planning was not only for the advancement of these colleagues but also for the continuation of the culture we had collectively developed.

Of course, I confronted the important grunt work of getting all the files in order, creating some summary files, especially on our history, and slowly emptying the spaces in my office for the new Chair. I was fortunate in the choice of the Chair of the search committee for my replacement.

> **Box 5.3 Announcement to Network Leaders and Department**
> After 22 years at Lehigh Valley Health Network, partnering with all of you to grow family medicine and primary care for our Lehigh Valley communities, I will be walking out of the Chair position as of mid-September of this year and walking into the next phase of my vocational adventure. I am not retiring as I have at least 3–4 more years of commitments on three national/international grants investigating primary care innovations and improvement and serving on the Board for the Society of Teachers of Family Medicine. I do plan to remain involved in teaching and mentoring and supporting Lehigh Valley Health Network where that could be helpful. How else I serve our larger vision of better health is still uncertain, but by celebrating abundance, mystery, and grace, I know the next steps will emerge over the next few months. In the meantime, LVHN has begun a national search process for a new Chair. But September is 9 months away, and we still have much to do, so we look forward to seeing each of you soon.

He was also a friend who spent extra time listening to department members and leaders and inviting me to meet key candidates and provide input. I wished for a new department chair who was younger, not quite ready for the role but with the right stuff, respect for the past, vision for the future, eager to tackle a growing network, and able to bring new strengths and gifts to the department. This plan reached fruition in their choice of Grant. My last day as Chair was October 12, 2016, with an official farewell reception on December 13, 2016 (see Box 5.4 for excerpts from my farewell comments). Midway through that year, it became clear to me that lingering on as an employed member of the department was not wise and would not reposition me or the department well for the future. I retired from employment on January 28, 2017.

> **Box 5.4 Farewell Comments Excerpts**
> - Almost 23 years ago, when I arrived in cold and deep, frozen snow and started in a trailer working with Headley White, Brian Stello, and Barbara Salvadore to begin family medicine here, I never anticipated what happened. Our intent was to build the best, most innovative community hospital family medicine residency and department in the country as a model for all and, in doing so, to help this place, my home for nine generations, become the healthiest place. Our purpose was to help Love grow. It's what

> we do here and who we have been. We aren't there yet, but we are surprisingly closer! Again, thank you!
> - We are, literally, at a watershed moment, transforming from serving the Lehigh River watershed to nearly all of the Delaware River watershed and more. Our passion for better medicine and our commitment to heal, comfort, and care for the people of our communities now extend to some of our region's most economically challenged areas. The scale and scope of our transformation will forever change us as an organization. But we cannot allow it to change our hearts and mission. Budget fears and, with such a grand scale, the inevitable tendency towards command and control will tug, but if we believe in each other and in our creativity, we can remain strong in our purpose.
> - When people fall into the muddiness of sickness, we are there offering what we in family medicine call turtle craft. We rise up from that mud, support our neighbors, and help them rejoin the living membership of their families and communities. It has been the greatest blessing to learn and serve with all of you, especially my turtle friends. Thank you! Keep watch, rise up, and be there, helping Love grow!

Part 2: Renewal

No sooner had the elevator doors closed behind me as I left One City Center than I was on my way to Belfast, Maine, to meet with two friends and so much more. Time for renewal and reimagining my vocation for the future. David, who breathed, lived, raised a family, and practiced his family medicine craft in Belfast for all his career, was considering retiring. Kurt, for whom the same was true but lived in Cleveland, Ohio, wanted to begin preparing for a retirement he now saw on the horizon. We were three family physician friends hoping to discover, "Now what?" as we approached leaving employment and shifting positions at this time in our lives and at this precarious time for our beautiful and broken earth that had gotten worse on our watch. We decided to create diverse inter-generational gatherings and conversations in each of our hometowns.

We began in Belfast, where David and Lindsey, who co-owned the local independent bookstore, welcomed Kurt and me into their home for 3 days. My son, Ethan, who also lives in Maine, was able to join us for one of those days. Exhilaration filled our hearts. David is deeply embedded and interwoven into the fabric of Belfast. Everyone knows him and has stories. We heard many, and we had extended conversations on belonging, the importance of tribe, helping in new ways and in different roles in the community, and supporting the next generations.

Just over 6 months later, in early August 2017, Kurt and David arrived at Deb's and my home in Allentown for 3 days of what I called "A gathering of crumbs, stones, and crows." Along with explorations of my ancestral home and local highlights and connections, we had a Sunday afternoon and an evening get-together with an inter-generational group of colleagues and a foraging format of numerous local, farm fresh, summer appetizers. We used a setup of multiple round tables to explore several topics including describing a generalist, relationship-centered healing craft in 2040 and describing leadership by elders living outside institutional power. In our conversations, we uncovered the dangers of persuasion and the power of hearing each other's stories. We reminded ourselves of the value of failure and the importance of elders supporting the young through them. The group especially helped me imagine how to transition from Chief to Tribal Elder. When we reconvened in the home of Kurt and Ann in Cleveland in late April 2018, these lessons were reinforced, and renewal seemed well underway, especially since my wife, Deb, had retired a month earlier to begin her own repositioning.

Meanwhile, Grant, the new family medicine chair at LVHN, assured me of a safe and wide passage into renewal. I was given a small office space, secretarial support, and emeritus medical staff status, which covered my malpractice costs thus allowing me to precept residents and teach medical students. I also retained my academic title as Professor of Family Medicine, which facilitated access to internal communications and library resources and smoothed research pathways. I continued to mentor, teach residents and medical students, and attend faculty meetings, and all on my own schedule. I maintained active research with my long-time best friend and research collaborator, Ben, and kept on enjoying winter cross-country ski adventures with fellow family physician leaders, Rob, Jeff, and Eric. The plan was working. Until it wasn't.

The heat of summer often finds a way to burn up my plans. In July, David decided to return to work as residency faculty and fellowship director in Bangor, and Kurt ramped up his leadership responsibilities and resumed grant writing in a big way. My friend, Ben, decided that retirement was years and years in the future, if ever. My resolve wavered a bit, and some self-doubt crept in. Minor blips, I told myself; my experiences as a tribal elder were going well. My plan left out my parents. In late August, my almost 94-year-old father suffered a stroke after a dental visit and never recovered, dying on September 12, 2 days before my birthday. My mother's chemotherapy-related mild dementia rapidly deteriorated over the next few months without his orienting presence, and she needed a transfer from her apartment to a memory care unit. My parents had a vacation place in the Poconos for over 70 years. My father also added to it every 5 years for 60 years, and what had been a little cabin in the woods was now significantly larger than my house. It was also crammed with 90 years of accumulated stuff. It took 2 years of steady effort to learn new and better ways of relating to my two siblings and to decumulate, repair, reminisce, grieve, celebrate, and ultimately sell the place. In between those spaces, I kept working the plan but trying to be a tribal elder for family medicine struggled to hold my attention.

I continued doing volunteer teaching, researching with Ben, seeing friends at conferences, skiing with Rob, Eric, and Jeff, and meeting with Kurt and David. Deb and I were able to do one of her dream vacations in late autumn 2018 to central Italy for cooking, picking olives, exploring history, and tasting wines. The following year, in September, we spent a month in France celebrating my 70th birthday with visits from Rob and Ben and their wives while investigating prehistoric cave art. But self-doubt and questions grew. I recognized the role of white male privilege that underlay my ability to do these things. Could I be doing more to address these disparities? In November, Ben found a melanoma on his foot. I learned of the deaths of three of my former longstanding patients and felt a twinge of betrayal at not being there for them and not being able to say goodbye. Three months later, the COVID-19 pandemic began. Losses were accumulating, and my plans evaporated. Whoa! Time to reset. Time to pay more attention to family and friends. Time to also pay more attention to inequity and the deteriorating condition of relational and generalist family medicine.

Part 3: Reset

What does it mean when you reposition and leave employment, but all your friends change their minds and don't? What happens when a global pandemic results in changes that dramatically alter what's possible and what's not? You reset. One of the core values of our residency program at Lehigh Valley is the celebration of abundance, mystery, and grace. It became my mantra.

The pandemic offered the gift of time and space and focused attention on family, friends, and the immediate life and people in front of me. Like the performers on Broadway, I left the stage and learned to work and thrive behind the scenes. No travel, no conferences, no going to the office to hang out with residents and faculty. Yes, virtual meetings substituted for these gatherings, but it wasn't the same. Then, as additional budget constraints frightened the network and they realized they owned too many buildings, they began downsizing office space. Appropriately, that included mine. They also converted emeritus medical staff status to more honorary and stopped paying for malpractice. For me, it meant the end of precepting or seeing patients in any capacity. Pappy's rocking chair came home.

Who was I now? Wrong question, I discovered. Who were Deb and I? Shifting to "we" revealed more abundant possibilities, humbled the ego, and opened wider to mystery and the likelihood that grace might happen. Rather than staring sadly at so many closed doors, we turned around to notice what else was there. We had gotten older, and our bodies knew it. Our minds were finally catching up. Grandparenting and our marriage moved to the center of attention. Deb and I began a more vigorous downsizing and decumulation and active exploration of future housing options. Our elementary school-age grandson, Loren, is homeschooled at his parents' farm collective in central Maine. Deb and I created a Salamander School of Wizardry taught by multiple spirit animals and aligned with his home school curriculum. He's been able to attend multiple two-week bursts of adventure, learning, loving, and memory-making for all three of us. All this activity of re-centering around home and family also helped me re-imagine my behind-the-scenes vocational identity.

I tightened connections with old friends. Fortunately, Ben's melanoma turned out to be local and resectable. We had often talked about a complete rewrite of our book, *Doing Qualitative Research*; however, he more seriously than I. We set about the researching and writing in earnest and finished the new edition. The flip side of my friends not retiring meant that they were all engaged in lots of stuff related to the present and future of family medicine. I was able to join them in those that especially fed my interests. Synergistically, this nourished our friendships. It also involved me in projects addressing the plight of generalist and relational primary medical care at the national and international levels.

Local mentoring relationships intensified, including supporting two projects focused on deepening connections and relationships between parts of the local healthcare systems and the more vulnerable communities that we serve. The first project engages multiple community groups and the local healthcare systems in addressing some of the maternal and child health issues affecting our neighbors lacking in social, environmental, and economic resources. Learning how to co-create a safe and trusting space for a group of community leaders, gang members, victims of abuse and violence, folks struggling with addiction, and healthcare professionals focuses the energies of the second project. Both, especially the latter, awaken hidden feelings and perspectives and open new possibilities, not only for the community but for my own growth. These experiences trouble the waters of one's self-understanding in healthy and profound ways. Both efforts are beginning to develop some momentum toward breaking down the barriers of privilege and closing many disparity gaps. I had led several similar initiatives in the past with little success. I discovered that quietly supporting others closer to the experiences generated more energy and agency.

I expanded my friendship network to include some persons I've admired from afar and wanted to know better. I joined an informal group named with the intent of bending the arc of history towards a better life together. Here were folks, family medicine leaders, who really did leave employment and were repositioning as tribal elders looking seven generations forward and searching out cracks in the dominating paradigm and seeking to widen them. We meet weekly, have published suggestions for a new kind of family medicine residency, and have started a website. Their examples and energy have been instrumental in helping me reset. And I connected with Lucy, resulting in this essay and this book.

Of course, with ageing, the losses accumulate. On April 20, 2021, my mom released her last exhalation as the final notes of Pachelbel's Canon in D faded into memory. She had been a guiding spirit in my life and the last of her generation in my family. I was now the family elder.

A reorientation happened. I, along with my wife, Deb, joined the council of tribal elders.

Part 4: Refresh

Come back, come home.
I'm gathering the crumbs and the stones.
Been travelling faster than my soul can go.
—Lyrics from chorus of Carrie Newcomer's "Speed of Soul"

Here we are 5 years after repositioning and walking away from employment. Very little is as we planned, but that's refreshing, and it feels good. Our daughter, Lindsay, has decided to leave the Lehigh Valley, where she has been most of her life, and move to northern Minnesota. No children of our family's next generation reside in the Lehigh Valley; Deb and I are among the last of ten generations in this place. We smile, in that enigmatic yet reassuring way that elders smile, and prepare for another major transition. Not planning as much and staying present more. Moments appear when memories of former patients linger, when I miss the excitement and rush of crises and decision-making and the joy of learning and discovery with faculty, residents, and students, and when I wish I had more new clinical stories and not just my old ones. But they happen much less often. Now I savor the moments when I listen to the younger generations share their stories, participate with Deb in making the ordinary in each day become extraordinary, openly appreciate the wonder in the eyes of our grandchild, take long walks along the Little Lehigh, and sprinkle a few crumbs, leave a few stones, and give voice with my fellow crows for the next seven generations. As the horizon of my life approaches, time concentrates.

Crumbs are what's left over after a fulfilling meal, the bits and scraps of sacred memories, like the tesserae of mosaics or the fragments and cut-outs that compose a scrapbook. We all accumulate these crumbs of wisdom that crumble around the messiness of our lives. Don't throw them away. Stones, on the other hand, remain after a building or wall collapses as remnants of foundations, still useful for their remembrances and for rebuilding. These are the stories that accrue. Preserve and use them with the crumbs. Crows eat the crumbs, watch over the stones, and store the stories and wisdom. Many cultures recognize crows as watchful, intelligent, clever, adaptable, vocal, loyal, magical thieves, and trickster sages. Working together, they serve as a symbol of change and transition, tribal elders of the living world. Repositioned, renewed, reset, and refreshed, Deb and I cherish becoming crows/elders as we gather the crumbs of wisdom from our lives and gather amidst the foundational stones and stories, letting go of the transitory trappings of success. We become present and act behind-the-scenes as tribal elders. The time may still come when our broken world or pained earth requires our presence on the front lines of protest. Be assured, we will rise with our aching bones and be there. We will gather the crumbs and the stones and our fellow crows and be home, moving at the speed of our souls. You are invited. Come, sit in Pappy's rocker (Fig. 5.1).

At least, that's the plan …

Fig. 5.1 Pappy's Rocker

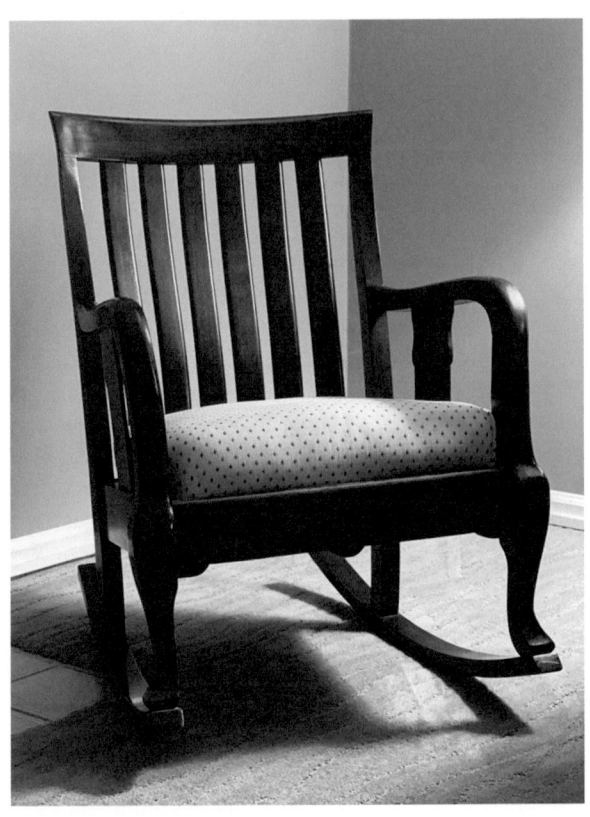

Chapter 6
A Stuttering Course to Retirement

Valerie J. Gilchrist

Editors' Introduction
When women in the Society of Teachers of Family Medicine (STFM) started to meet together without men in hotel rooms where the annual conferences were held, Valerie Gilchrist was one of the first people to arrive. She was clear from early in her career that women faculty in family medicine had more roles and more challenges than our male colleagues and that the organization of faculty family physicians needed to recognize their needs with childcare arrangements at meetings, breastfeeding locations, and time for meeting separately as a special interest group or committee. Equity in leadership, plenary speakers, and program content began to transform the organization. Valerie Gilchrist emerged as a leader in the group that pushed the strong women's focus in STFM meetings over the 80s and 90s with many women leaders emerging and challenging the still largely male-dominated leadership of departments of family medicine. Not surprisingly, Val became a feminist chair of family medicine in three different departments over the course of her career and continues to draw attention to the ongoing forces limiting women's advancement. Widely recognized as an organizational leader, educator, and editor, Val is a skilled collaborator, always mentoring her more junior colleagues in their writing and research while supporting strategies for their successful combination of clinical work, teaching, and parenting and partnering, adding academic achievement when ready.

As she describes in her essay, Val carved her own kind of feminism; doing her life and work the way she wanted was her kind of feminism. But, as she points out, as an initial woman leader in the places where she was Chair, the path was a lonely one. She cultivated her feminist colleagues in other disciplines and in other geographies, often travelling to connect with her distant peers. Retirement will open the

---

V. J. Gilchrist (✉)
Department of Family Medicine and Community Health, University of Wisconsin, Madison, WI, USA
e-mail: Valerie.gilchrist@fammed.wisc.edu

opportunity for her to enjoy friends and family in her native Canada, where her longest-time feminist friends await her visits. Our loss will be their gain.

This is a meandering story of retirement coming into focus. I was never one to set my 5-year goals, not really even my 1-year goal. I can set direction, yes, but goals always seemed fallacious. I know what I'd like to get done this week, but next week may present something different.

I didn't set a date for "retirement." Thinking of retirement was both a statement of longing and of evasion. Retirement happened to other people. I could not imagine it for myself. Part of that is me, and part of that is the profession of medicine. I vividly remember when someone told me I did not have the right work-life balance. That I worked all the time and that, as a leader, I was sending the wrong message to others. I was furious. How dare you tell me how I should live my life? I have the work-life balance that works for me. It is not the same as it was when I entered practice, not the same as when my children were small, not the same as it was 10 years ago or even 1 year ago, and not the same as it will be next year and the year after. It is constantly changing as I change and the situation and the people who are important to me change. I think of retirement or transitions in the same way. What works for me may not work for you.

My depression-era father, who got his engineering degree on war bonds after WWII, and my British mother, who lost her first husband in WWII and lived through "the Blitz," brought to my sister and me the unspoken belief that like, the Ralph Waldo Emerson quote, "The purpose of life is not to be happy. It is to be useful…." My parents highly regarded independence and work that made a difference. I recall my father telling me explicitly that I needed to have a career so "I would never have to depend on a man to take care of me." My work is not something I do. It is who I am and what I can contribute to this life.

Major transitions in my adult life were based not on meeting a set goal but rather on both the slowly accumulating gifts of reflection and moments of absolute assurance—when what turned out to be life-altering decisions were right for me.

Initial Thoughts: "This Is Paramedic Joe"

On June 21, 2018, to this day, I can smell the *pho* and hear paramedic Joe's voice. I had just entered the kitchen carrying dinner. My phone went off, and the screen showed my husband's name. I answered, "Hi, Honey," and the response was, "This is paramedic Joe." My husband Bill had been performing with his band in 'Make Music Madison,' an annual event on the summer solstice during which musicians, professionals, and amateurs perform free for the public. The band had just finished; they stood to take a bow, and then Bill recalls no more until he became aware of someone pounding on his chest. The paramedic was explaining what had happened and asked repeatedly if I was "alright." Of course, I understood what had happened; I could see it all too vividly. I remember trying very hard not to scream back, "For God's sake stop talking to me and get him to the (expletive) ED!" Morgaine, our daughter, still standing holding the *pho*, numbly followed me to the car to drive the 25 min to the hospital. I used my badge and went directly into the ED, to the large trauma bay, and then stopped short. It was quiet. The doors were wide open, only a nurse starting clean up. I took in the detritus of the code—alcohol swabs on the floor still pink, an occasional gauze pad, carts askew, and Bill lying flat on the bed in the center of the room, not moving. He looked so white, like his gray hair and the bed sheets. He looked stunned, staring up at the ceiling. He knew me and weakly smiled.

The combination of his performing in a public park with an AED (automated external defibrillator), someone in the audience who knew how to use it, the fire station two blocks away, and the university hospital 2 miles away resulted in him getting his three stents and an ICD (implantable cardioverter defibrillator) within an hour of his collapse. Bill is now fine although complaining of all the pills he takes.

An event like this put the reality of our limited lifespan squarely in front of me. Bill was retired. We have been married for 47 years. I began then saying to myself "How much longer do I want to work?" I need to make time now for things we want to do.

A Career Trajectory

I did not set out to be a department chairperson, although I have held chair positions for the majority of my career. I wanted to be a clinician and a small-town family doctor like the one I grew up with. However, after following Bill to his new tenure-track position in the United States, I found myself in northern Ohio at the time that a new medical school opened. I then discovered I enjoyed teaching, research, and the little bit of administration that came with directing the school's Office of Women in Medicine while my clinical practice grew exponentially. What happened? How did I become a Chair—by default! Our new Department Chair did not show up for the first day of work. Truly, the welcome banner was hanging when the Dean received the email in which the candidate said he could not take the job. This caused much consternation, talks about a new search, and then the decision to approach local program leaders. I don't know how many others were approached, but when I was asked, I said "Yes" because I knew absolutely, "Someone has to do this job." And I could work hard. I could be of use in the career I loved and with my peers.

Working in northern Ohio for 17 years before becoming a Chair, I practiced full-scope family medicine, developed friendships, and had three children. I learned how to be a clinician. For the 8 years I was Chair, I learned about what one person can and cannot accomplish in a regional medical school. In 2005, I was frustrated, and our family stage offered possibilities. It was time to learn again in another type of medical school. Our eldest had left for university, our second was going the next year, our youngest was ready to enter middle school, and my husband had an upcoming sabbatical.

The timing was right, and although I knew I would be taking on even more, I found this change to be harder than my first move, even though that first move was across national borders. It was less of an exciting adventure than one of recognizing losses as I moved. What about the responsibility of moving my family? The move to the USA 25 years prior was for Bill's job. Now I was the one causing disruption for our family. It was an exciting move for me, but what about the others in our family? Was I being selfish? And would I find new friends, both personal and professional? And most worrisome was, what about my patients, some of whom had been driving an hour to see me? I can still feel the very long "saying goodbye" visits. There were young mothers whom I'd delivered, and both of us were shedding tears. I realized that no one else might ever know the secrets of a particular four-generation family I served. I held tightly the only copy of the recipe for her Italian wedding cake that my patient said had ever gone out of the family. I was losing the many loving relationships with patients that daily restored me much more than their care drained me. I would miss that sustenance.

In my short 3 years at East Carolina University, Brody School of Medicine, the school experienced a near financial collapse. I worked with perhaps the most dedicated group of clinicians caring for the most underserved population I had ever known and began to appreciate how innovation in family medicine can impact a healthcare system. I had had no intention of leaving, but when the University of Wisconsin (UW) came looking, and as it became more and more apparent that my husband was not happy, the next move was absolutely clear.

My 12 years as Chair at UW were challenging, energizing, and ultimately overwhelming. In retrospect, although I was a good leader at first, I did not learn to manage and lead this large department well enough to satisfy me and the team of amazing clinicians and staff. My energy and joy started to decrease, and my anxieties increased in the year after Bill had his "event." The constant worry about missing an important email, and feeling as if I never had the time to really talk to people, or plan strategically, were subsumed in what felt like a daily crush of never-ending things to do.

Reflections on "Being Driven"

I have felt driven by external demands, children, patients, and deadlines but also by the incessant internal demand of myself that I could be and should be better than I was, and do more than I did. Feeling driven had a real everyday cadence that, although faded now, was a fact of everyday life. There were always "things to do" with a full-scope family medicine academic practice and three children and a working spouse and no family nearby or live-in help. Who is going to pick up which child? Who is going to take them to whatever activity? Who has an evening or travel commitment? Who is making dinner? It was a tightly choreographed dance that now I wish had not been so stressful, especially for our children. However, being internally driven is something else.

Being driven to excel in work was absorbed from my childhood ethos of work being one's purpose in life. Full-scope family medicine can be all-encompassing. Work could win out over family, friends, or personal happiness, a socially rewarded characteristic for a physician. I am certainly not alone among physicians who put work first. We know how to be workers. Great to have in your doctor but not maybe so great in a friend or parent or partner… or at a dinner party. I can laugh now but truly was shocked years ago to overhear an acquaintance telling another friend about the horribly boring party she had recently attended with no one there but boring doctors. I found myself thinking about my doctor friend parties. Yes, we all left early because we were sleep-deprived. Yes, we talked about what was most important to us, our work. Was that a statement of values, or was it simply that we knew nothing else? This reinforces the isolation of physicians. Do we know no other way of being with others other than as a doctor?

This "work first" priority was exacerbated by my feeling that I had to prove myself as a female and as a family physician. My medical school class in Canada was almost 20% female, but I started practicing in the US because it was Bill's turn to choose, and there were few women. Family medicine was an underappreciated specialty. In my first year of practice, a consulting urologist said to me, "Valerie, I didn't use to like women doctors, but you're different." He meant that as a compliment.

I was the only woman clinical department Chair in my first and second Chair positions. In my third, there was one other female Chair (in pediatrics), and in the next year, a third came. Why do I mention this? Because the work that took most of my waking hours was lonely. I came into my second and third Chair positions as an outsider and could not develop friendships with those in my department. The prior male Chair recommended my friendships be with my fellow Chairs, but those were all white, mostly older men, not my peer group. I just worked harder—alone.

I also wanted very much for our Department of Family Medicine to innovate and make a difference. Why could not the Universities understand how good Family Medicine and Primary Care could improve care for the population? The cynic in me says it's because "they" did not care. That of course is not true, but rather that, individually, none of them could fight the dysfunctional US healthcare system. Although the capacity at UW was inspiring, even the little pieces of improving care locally I found difficult.

I felt I should be opening paths for future women in medicine, promoting the stature of Family Medicine in a traditional University, and developing a department that could lead national change for the social good. Writing that makes me realize even more of my hubris. I was critical of myself and others. I was burning out. Burnt out and dysfunctional. Isolating myself. I did not take stock of what I should do or ask for help from others, but I talked to the Dean and announced that I would be stepping away from the Chair position in July 2019. But after just 4 months, in a moment of absolute clarity, I called the Dean to tell him I needed to step away from the Chair position at that time. The Dean knew I was emotionally done and did not try to dissuade me.

I am so much a happier person. The weight of expectations is gone. My energy and laughter and time for friends have increased. For me, the time was right. I wondered if I would miss being "in the know," but I don't miss it at all. It feels wonderful not to feel responsible for everything. Now I am doing a little research and more clinical work. My pace of life and joy have changed.

Now that I could do things other than work, especially administrative work, I feel like a different person. I feel like me, not the Chair me. Is this returning to my "authentic self"? I don't think so. My authentic self is both what I was in the past and what I am becoming for the future. I do know, however, that I am a happier person.

The Pandemic and Returning to Clinical Medicine

My transition from being the Chair coincided with the pandemic. Everybody's job changed at that time. I began to do more clinical work because it was needed. I could back up in the clinic for others called to the hospital. I could do telemedicine. Clinical work not only filled the void for me but also gave me back my sense of meaning. Now that the pandemic is at a different stage, roles are changing. I can continue to provide clinical care as much as I want. However, how much do I want? Where do I fit?

At my clinical office, our rural teaching site 20 miles from Madison, I am a known quantity. I was never really the Chair there. I was another doctor who was in and out and had her patient panel. I feel comfortable there. I am also now an "in house locum" going where I'm needed. Nonetheless, I really don't quite fit. I am not core resident faculty. I don't fit in research without a research team or external funding. I am that person who can be called on to represent the department on the most tedious and inconsequential university committee. I understand that what is implicit, if not explicit, is 'but how long will you be here?'

What do you do with a previous Chair who is on an undefined job and an unknown trajectory to retirement? I no longer have administrative support, a substantial shock after 27 years. I don't fit within our compensation package. A former faculty member whom I helped attain tenure is our current Chair. Discussing my plans with me, he looks worried as we review the department challenges. I recognize his worry about resources. I know that my costs are not growing a future but honoring a past. There is little room for that in a departmental budget. It is awkward for both of us. I'm glad he is a kind, smart man whom I like and who is trustworthy and honest. We are both in unexplored territory. I tell him my tentative plans. He accepts them. We will revisit this in another 6 months.

As I stepped away from administration to do more clinical work, I realized there were limitations, both physical and mental. Neither my body nor my mind are as agile as they once were. Through 2020, I agreed to cover the night/weekend call schedule for the person who took on the role of interim Chair. I had given up OB after 25 years in 2005, and in 2021 I stopped call and inpatient medicine. Although

I then felt as if I were half a physician, I also knew that the sleep disruption of calls in the middle of the night drained me. I also wondered if I was adding anything substantive to residents' nighttime decisions.

I could liberate myself of administrative responsibilities and delightfully give up call and inpatient work, but would I give up my patients? Patient care is not the burden of administrative responsibilities I carried, but rather it is the well-worn cloak I have worn as soft as skin. "You're not going to retire yet are you?" my patients ask me not infrequently. Their worry is affirming, yet I know I am slower. I have been a family physician for 45 years. That means years and years of gifts such as hand-crafted mementos, baby blankets, fresh produce, and more amazing baking than I could eat in a lifetime. It means joining families in moments of joy and grief, relationships ripening like fine wine and most intimate, pats on my hand of a said and unsaid statement, "I love you" and "I love you too." I am so fortunate to have received these overwhelming gifts of friendship and trust. It humbles me. I am so grateful. I want to send a letter of thanks to my patients on retirement, not the health system's notice of retirement. I want to say, "Thank you," and that it is because I cherish you, my patients, that I need to retire. You need someone who is "on the top of it" all the time. Who is, yes, younger and smarter, to take care of you.

When I left my practice in Ohio, I left to start work in another practice. When I give up my clinical license and my patients this time, I will be leaving forever. What will it be like leaving this core part of my identity? What will I be? I have squeezed, tried to open, and rubbed repeatedly at this purpose. I know that clinical life is still a part of who I am, but it is not all of who I am. I am changing a way of being in this world that makes room for other ways of being. I will always be a family doctor, a mother, a wife, a reader, a writer, a friend, and who else knows what!

A Delight in Slowing Down … Allowing Time with the Trivial

I don't run anymore; I walk. I try to make it a brisk walk, but my Apple watch puts me solidly in the 20-min mile club. So much for speed! Physically, everything is stiffer, and I don't push myself as much as I used to. I want only some muscle ache. If I walk too far for too long, my hip aches. I know I should return to the morning weight class at 0530, but the zest for being up in the dark is gone.

And yes, I am slowing down mentally. It was those little black things… that are very salty; … I wanted to add them to the lemon pasta…. Oh yes, capers! How is it that words hide behind my thoughts for no reason? It is especially embarrassing when it is a name, and I can't get away with "your son" or some such slide.

I am somewhat surprised that I am quite fine with slowing down. No longer the person who could get everything done, I am deliciously sliding into another lifestyle. I read or talk to family or even, heaven forbid, watch television in the evening. I read email other than in bed at night and am almost keeping up reading some journals. I so enjoy reading more books, a delight that I usually lost to sleep in the past. Now I can have both. I find joy in the momentary exquisite observations of the day—the clouds, the quiet, the smell of ripe tomatoes, the bird songs, the wind—most of which I had not even had the presence of mind to dismiss. What a gift!

We used to have what my mother called "lovelies," fine porcelain with hand-painted gilt edges, a hand-woven table piece bursting with color that was a wedding present, a wood picture crafted so one can see the wind blowing. And I am having such fun giving them away. I am done with things. I'm not dying, or at least not that I know of, at least not soon, but those figurines need to be enjoyed and not just catching dust. Others can feel gratitude and wonder at the talent and work of these artists. Our children don't want all of them, but others do. They should be loved, as I am and we are, in the shrinking down part of our lives.

I am becoming more and more conscious of the limited time I have in this life to do the things I really love. We lost two of our contemporary group of friends, and one of my dearest friends had a stroke this past spring. I wonder who is next. Although I love my work as a physician and I so enjoy time with my patients, I can ask myself what I really want to do now. Not tomorrow, when the "work" has been done.

Decision

I enjoy travel and there are so many places yet to see. It was very challenging for me to be separated from many of our close friends and my family during the pandemic. The place I love most in the world is our shared lodge on a river system in Ontario. We had gone every year since 1979 except for the summer of 2020. This is my 'soul place.' I want more time to enjoy it. We finally bought the boat that we've loved and been talking about buying for over a decade. This past summer it became clear to me at the lodge that I need not finish this or that project, that **I** was the limiting factor for my retirement. It is true that I have provided our major income, and it would be disingenuous of me not to mention money. However, when sitting at the Lodge, I was finally able to make peace with the knowledge that there will never be enough money to totally relieve my anxieties **and** accept that there will always be sufficient money. There will also be enough time to worry about money when I don't remember how to worry. Most important now is the time for every day, sleeping in until the sun comes up, snuggling with Bill watching silly shows and the occasional fine movie, and more and more laughing with friends. I want to visit my adult children on a whim. I am absolutely sure it is now time to stop the slide to retirement and set the date.

My retirement date is now set. Full retirement—walk out the door, hand over the coded cards, stop renewing my medical licenses or keeping up with CME, and move to emerita status. The picture snapped into place. It feels so exciting, even though there are still many decisions to be made. We need to continue to "give away" items. I am Canadian; Bill is American. We have family in both countries. We will spend time with all. It is time to do more of what I love most. It is time for self-compassion, living in the moment with gratitude and faith in the future.

Chapter 7
For the Curious: A Brief Literature Review

Lucy M. Candib

Editors' Introduction

A hefty literature concerning retirement exists. But when you begin to enter more keywords like "medicine," "physicians," and "family medicine," the bulk of the pile significantly lessens. Add "leaving relationships," and the number of references almost disappears. Using a question-and-answer format and the keywords noted, here's what Lucy discovered.

Why Do Doctors Depart from Practice?

Doctors have to say goodbye for a variety of reasons: finishing residency or fellowship, a better job elsewhere for the doctor or his/her spouse, emerging new priorities in career focus or practice type, serious illness for the doctor or his/her spouse that requires realigning the family's priorities, life cycle changes for the doctor such as multiple demands of children and/or aging parents, and finally retirement. Retirement from clinical work is a specific challenge for the doctor because it potentially means an end to the intellectual and relational activities that brought satisfaction, pleasure, and status, along with substantial financial reward to the doctor, often over many years.

L. M. Candib (✉)
Family Medicine and Community Health, University of Massachusetts Chan Medical School, Worcester, MA, USA

If Retirement Is a "Problem," What Is the Solution?

The literature focusing on retirement for physicians typically offers recommendations on the personal aspects of retirement. Some articles are short "how to" primers that address the importance of advance planning: how to maintain financial stability, how to negotiate new roles in the household, and then the importance of planning one's time, especially for those physicians for whom medicine was their "whole life"—those who did not have "outside interests." In other words, retirement for physicians seemed to be a problem, yet the "treatment" consisted of a hodgepodge of "tips" for success. Some academic physicians see the departure from medical institutions as leading to such a serious loss of status and collegial connections that they choose not to retire—they can't imagine professional life outside the institutions of power where they have been powerful figures. A 2016 systematic review of reasons for physician retirement drew the following expectable conclusion:

> Excessive workload and burnout were frequently cited reasons for early retirement. Ongoing financial obligations delayed retirement, while strategies to mitigate career dissatisfaction, workplace frustration, and workload pressure supported continuing practice [1].

Later retirement was associated with physicians' strong sense of value of their work and the desire to maintain the cognitive and social aspects of practice.

What About Younger Physicians?

A typical time when physicians leave patients is at the end of their residency. Here again, the focus is on how to *do it* in such a way that patients have smooth transitions to their new clinicians. The importance of this comes up in the educational recommendations on how to teach residents to go through the process of thoughtfully and respectfully ending relationships with patients with adequate planning for them and their patients to say their goodbyes. A study of a unique educational program to prepare pediatric residents for leaving their practice and leaving their patients had what appeared to be surprising results: residents were unaware of which patients had strong attachments, and they themselves had strong attachments to their preceptors, office staff, and patients as well. In other words, the doctors' emotional responses to the separation and losses involved in leaving a practice are usually hidden from view; in fact, at times it appears that doctors are trained not to think that their feelings (when they can acknowledge them) are relevant to the process.

Has Medicine Paid Much Attention to Ending Clinical Relationships?

Even in the educational setting, most of the attention paid to saying goodbye and transferring patients has addressed the instrumental aspects of patient treatment: when and how to tell patients, arranging the mechanics of the transfer of care, and even planning for the challenges of telling dependent or needy patients about the doctor's impending departure. The intensity of this process seemed to have come as a surprise to the pediatric residents studied [2], perhaps because the role of the doctor-patient relationship had not been central in their training. Another pediatric residency assessed residents' emotions at the end of their third year and found relief but also sadness, guilt, and worry over the fear of abandonment of patients. These themes get little attention in most of today's training programs [3]. Doctors looking at their feelings is not a strong suit in much of medical education.

What About When Retirement Is the Reason for the Doctor's Departure?

More recently, physician retirement finally became a focus of academic interest. The main systematic review of this literature by Silver et al. [1] looked at when physicians retire, why they retire early, why some delay retirement, and how institutions might best enable physicians to work longer or plan their withdrawal from the work setting more successfully. In fact, the meaning of retirement for physicians had not been carefully examined. Let's look at what has been considered: the doctors' personal experience of leaving their lifelong careers and the institutional considerations.

What Might Be the Meanings of Retirement for Men and Women Doctors Toward the End of Their Careers?

For some, retirement could clearly serve as an identity threat [4]. When professionals in late careers maintain a single-minded vision of what constitutes success, they may have more difficulty considering retirement as an option and in accepting the "diversification" that is necessary for a successful retirement. Here, the loss of identity that comes with physician retirement was interpreted as a need to take up new kinds of interests if they hadn't existed before. Put another way, the possibility of "reimagining the self" would mean creating meaning through new activities and finding another way to live and give through the family and grandchildren [5]. Women in academic medicine may have a different transition to and concept of retirement. Because, for women, the harmonizing of family and profession has usually been a goal and at least a partial accomplishment throughout their careers [6], later career choices may not be so problematic [5].

What's the Impact on Institutions of Physician Retirement?

The retirement of their most experienced and skilled physicians has been a perennial problem for academic medical centers. After conducting focus groups about later life transitions with academic physicians in Canada, Silver et al. [7]

recommended that the institutions themselves "support flexible, agentive, and respectful retirement transitions" as a way to balance both the needs of those considering retirement and the institutional needs for recruitment and retention.

Medical academia may, however, set up its own complications. Over the years, full-time work in some settings may have been incompatible with composing a life that included more than work, or any consideration of today's shorthand version, "work-life balance," leading senior physicians not to seriously consider retirement, as their identity was/is completely linked with their work. In contrast, nowadays, younger generations may choose differing priorities and see the older generation as refusing to cede territory for promotion. The senior generation may view the younger generation as less dedicated to the work. The institutions may not recognize this conflict and continue to avoid facilitating transitions for both generations that might have more harmonious and perhaps healthier strategies both for individuals and for institutions [8]. These conclusions came from a detailed qualitative study of numerous academic physicians in a large department of internal medicine in Toronto and may not generalize to retirement decisions in other settings, particularly primary care, and to other institutions and nations with differing approaches to financing retirement, promoting part-time transitions, and fostering well-being in the older age group. Women physicians who have successfully found ways to merge "part-time" work (even up to 40 h) with childbearing, parenting, self-care, and family life over the past few decades may view the transition to retirement much less negatively and feel less conflicted about retirement than previous generations and, in particular, the academic physicians in Silver's study [8].

What Might Recommendations for "Flexible, Agentive, and Respectful Retirement Transitions" [7] Mean?

Potentially, these late career transitions might include the possibility of taking up or maintaining certain kinds of non-clinical roles in medicine. For instance, mentoring, teaching, and volunteering can allow for limited but rewarding roles that don't bring with them the pressured weight of unrewarding administrative tasks such as charting and billing. Onyura et al. suggest that the retiring academic physician can develop a "diversified portfolio of selves" that allows the physician retiring from seeing patients to find psychosocial rewards outside of clinical practice and to maintain "resilience in the face of identity threats that manifest when one plans (or is forced) to discontinue work" [4, p. 289].

What Happened to the Relationships in all This Retirement Talk?

For the most part, the small literature on retirement issues fails to address the loss of relationships. The family medicine literature in particular does not usually address this loss directly but instead offers anecdotes. Most first-person descriptions of retirement or departure are in medicine's "occasional literature" or what Medline calls "Anecdotes as Topic"—essays, narratives, and "Life's Stories" [9–11]. For instance, Peter Curtis writes about finding himself signing personal letters to 600 patients during a snowstorm that brought home to him the "swirling memories of the interlocking problems, relationships, and triumphs of families" for whom he had been the personal doctor [9, p. 573].

An occasional retired physician writes about getting more satisfaction from the doctoring they do after retirement compared to before. Renate Justin felt sad and "dispirited" following her retirement from general practice after 50 years, thinking that she would no longer be able to "comfort and heal" [12]. Nevertheless, she found that neighbors and friends and some former patients contacted her and even came to her home for what she could offer: her ability to listen. And in some cases, she was called upon to work her magic—for instance, she was asked to go to the hospital to convince a confused former patient to get undressed, as neither doctors nor nurses were able to convince the woman to disrobe. Other retirees find specific niches where they can continue doing valuable clinical work, but in a time- and responsibility-limited way. For instance, cardiologist Lawrence Hergott, after retiring from his "lifelong dream," found his way to do one-time cardiology consultations for primary care doctors in a large cardiology group with an access problem; he reports "having a blast" seeing patients in one-off consultation visits [11].

So, Is Saying Goodbye Really Hard?

Yes, it actually is! Saying goodbye to patients in primary care (and in other specialties with a focus on chronic care where long-term relationships have been common) is a challenging problem for doctors in multiple dimensions. Leaving cherished relationships with individuals and families that have lasted decades and even an adult patient's entire lifetime is a great loss for both doctors and patients [13]. Additionally, leaving staff and colleagues who have been long-term companions in clinical work in various settings is also a source of emotional loss [2]. Surprisingly, the literature on retirement for physicians mostly avoids the feelings of loss provoked by these departures, a denial of grief. The literature on how to "manage" leaving clinical practice (for whatever reason—retirement, career transition, or relocation) mostly avoids the emotional aspect of leaving. Boekelheide [13] is a very early exception to such avoidance in the family medicine literature. In contrast, Lucy's and Eydie's story about the retirement of a family doctor from long-term practice (see Chap. 8) is a story about the loss of caring relationships with patients—in other words, looking at retirement from a relational perspective.

What About Other Family Doctors' Experience of Loss?

Other family doctors who might readily admit, in person, a deep feeling of loss about stopping or scaling back practice only comment on it indirectly in print. David Loxterkamp [14], writing a "Eulogy" for his vocation, talks about his sensation that his personal calling was "slipping away," when he and his colleague scaled down their practice and eliminated hospital medicine from the "doctor's work." But his grief here was more for the loss of his vision or dream of his identity rather than the loss of relationships, since, in his transition, relationships with patients may well have deepened as, afterward, he spent more time with patients in the office or with former patients in the community. In another example, when the Merensteins examined the communications from 200 patients on the occasion of Joel Merenstein's retirement after 43 years of practice, they analyzed only the themes from the patients' letters. Regarding *his* feelings about leaving so many cherished relationships, they mentioned, only as a "bias," their adherence to the Balint principle: "the desire by the physician to be perceived positively and even loved by these people and sadness and guilt at leaving them" [15, p. 462]. But they did not explore that "sadness and guilt," nor what he himself would miss about those many relationships.

Was There an Occasional Explicit Recognition of Loss?

Recognition has, however, seeped out anecdotally of the family doctor avoiding facing the emotional aspect of his/her departure. For example, when Ann C. Macaulay was leaving a community of 5000 people in Quebec after 18 years, a patient who was also a colleague, after a miscarriage, started crying and blurted out to Macaulay, "I don't know what I am grieving the most—the loss of this baby or the loss of you." At that point, Macaulay herself started to cry and recalls: "I will always be grateful to her. Until then, I had been very objective about the problems my patients were having, but she helped me understand that I too was grieving" [10, p. 64]. Sometimes it takes a supportive setting for the physician's feelings to emerge. In an academic article advocating for the role of Balint groups for physicians leaving practice, the leader pushed a clinician to recognize her avoidance of patients' feelings due to her own sense of loss in leaving a treasured practice. In this context, the group members could recognize that "patients and their doctors are attached through subtle, usually unspoken threads" [16, p. 551].

What About Other Specialties? Do They Address the Loss of Relationship When Doctors Move or Retire?

Specialists who have long-term relationships with seriously ill patients no doubt have such experiences when they make career changes, but their explicit public acknowledgement of loss is also rare. One impressive exception to this omission is an unusual book co-authored by a patient with connective tissue disease and demyelinating neuropathy, Alida Brill, and her doctor, an academic rheumatologist, Michael D. Lockshin: *Dancing at the River's Edge: A Patient and Her Doctor Negotiate Life with Chronic Illness* [17]. In a chapter revealingly titled "Interdependence: The Doctor Moves to NIH," Lockshin writes about his experience of leaving his academic practice at a New York City specialty center and moving to Washington in the hopes of influencing national health policy. He writes eloquently of his aching pain, leaving behind his patients. After talking of his own family, he writes:

> But what of the other family, the patients whose lives are intertwined with mine, from whom I would now take leave? ... there were tears–on both sides–and an attempt to arrange ongoing care. And moments of anguish: some patients were very sick (Alida among them) and I did not want to leave them to another's care [17, p. 138].

> I did not lose the sense that I had abandoned those who were most desperately ill. In my practice life I had not run from the bedside of someone whom I could no longer save [17, p. 140].

For Lockshin, *being there* and *being with* are central to his understanding of the clinical relationship. Within nursing, this phrase is considered central to the concept of presence, a necessary way of being in nursing practice with patients [18]. Here was a doctor who, through his long-term relationships with chronically ill patients, often through multiple crises and hospitalizations, could acknowledge the depth and length of his own sense of loss brought about by his choice to depart.

Most doctors, family doctors and specialists, never talk about termination, retirement, or job change the way that Lockshin does. It takes a brave clinician to acknowledge how much pain we have caused both to our patients and to our own selves when the life-changing decisions we have made provoke such intense feelings of loss for both parties. For the clinician, this experience is multiplied over and over again with each patient and his or her family, usually during the same few months.

What About Psychiatry? Do Psychiatrists Address Their Feelings of Loss?

Psychoanalysis is the one area of medicine where saying goodbye, in the form of "termination," takes on a life of its own, which I will address in a moment. Yet family medicine is unlike psychoanalysis, where the whole point of the work is paradoxical: "to foster an intimacy that intends separation" [19]. Family medicine, in fact, maintains its cradle-to-grave imagery, although it is always the patients whose cradles and graves are intended, not the doctor's. The doctor's ending of the relationship is the antithesis of this sometimes mythical version of family medicine.

How Does the End of the Relationship Between Patient and Physician Compare Between Family Medicine and Psychiatry?

The family medicine engagement with the individual and, hopefully, part or all of the nuclear family and sometimes beyond, depending on the size of the community, shares the very long commitment across the lifespan of both patient and doctor. Psychoanalysis is also a very long-term commitment as well, sometimes measured in decades but usually having an end called termination—the planned ending or goal of successful "analysis." Termination has been a highly charged subject dating back to Freud and continuing even today as a topic of concern and even debate [20]. But interestingly enough, even when psychiatrists address the challenges of termination, it is mostly the patient whose complicated feelings (resistance, anger, regression, and hostility) are to be explicitly interpreted and managed. The occasional mention of the countertransference (the therapist's response to the patient's words, actions, and feelings) historically mostly omits explicit acknowledgment of the affective component of this work—the anger, loss, and grief of the loss of caring relationships often lasting many years—which, though unmentioned, may still simmer underneath the professional stance. A 2008 panel on termination did address the psychiatrist's own feelings, of his/her countertransference, to be analyzed but not discussed, and not viewed as appropriate for expression either to the patient, or even to colleagues, unless very problematic. That the analyst goes through such a distinct process of mourning at the end of a patient's analysis was acknowledged in that panel as a particularly difficult time [20].

Judith Viorst, a non-physician analyst probably best known for her authorship of *Alexander and the Terrible, No-Good, Very Bad Day*, recognized the startling lack of information about how analysts manage this challenge of loss after ending analyses and interviewed 20 psychoanalysts, under the cloak of anonymity, about their personal reactions to the end of long-term treatment with their patients [21]. She reports that in the interviews, each of them "made a serious effort at self-examination … and that because of the isolation of their work, they found pleasure and relief in talking about it" [21, p. 401]. These interviews confirm that most psychiatrists do experience, but never overtly acknowledge, deep feelings of sadness and loss with the closure of long-term clinical relationships. She found that some analysts identified how they had used a patient's termination "to resolve some piece of their own unfinished business" [21, p. 417]. Her conclusion is that "the need to identify, resolve, and digest one's losses is a significant technical issue for the psychoanalyst during the terminal phase … that in dealing with aspects of loss, analysts may find that they can utilize their responses for their own–as well as their patients'–further development" [21, p. 400]. Viorst quotes Michael Balint with regard to termination:

> It is a deeply moving experience; the general atmosphere is of taking leave forever of something very dear, very precious—with all the corresponding grief and mourning … .Usually the patient leaves after the last session happy but with tears in his eyes and … I think I may admit---the analyst is in a very similar mood [22, p. 197].

Balint had historically worked with medical doctors in Hungary before emigration to Great Britain with his wife and colleague Enid Balint in 1939 and went on to work with British family doctors in formation of what we now know as Balint groups. So Balint offers a significant link to the importance of the work of saying goodbye at the end of long-term relationships in both psychiatry and in family medicine.

Are There any Narratives Co-written by Clinicians and Patients?

The alternating chapters in Lockshin's and Brill's narrative on the course of Brill's illness and its complications provide a moving panorama of a very long-term clinical relationship treasured by both. Not surprisingly, as they co-wrote this book, they became increasingly good friends who trusted and respected each other. Another co-written narrative that resulted in a deep friendship is *The Light Within* [23], in which a physician who was a fellow in gynecologic oncology (Lois Ramondatta) met a woman beginning her cancer treatment (Debra Sills). Lois' clinical involvement with Debra was brief, but their personal relationship evolved through the last years of Debra's life as they worked on their co-written (in alternating voices) narrative describing the concurrent development of their friendship, the growing connection between their families, their deepening understandings of what a living and dying person needs, and the ultimately inevitable, unrelenting course of Debra's disease.

Collaborating on writing books and essays about the process both doctor and patient have experienced not surprisingly transforms the relationship from a series of clinical interactions into a different kind of joint project, and in both of these instances, a deep friendship was the result. Another language to describe this is offered by Arthur Frank, who might call the alternating narrative a "companion story." He proposes that "any relation of care is a dialogical process: each comes to speak in the voice of the other, shaping and being shaped by the other" [24, p. 126].

Does the Perspective of Autoethnography Have Anything to Offer Clinicians Thinking About Considering Retirement?

The process of paying attention to and writing about retirement can also be viewed from a research perspective called autoethnography—a way of documenting for others a person's own self-reflection in a way that tries to situate the experience in a broader social and political context. It is a kind of qualitative research that allows the exploration of personal vulnerability for the purpose of revealing the broader dynamics at work in a family, an organization, a culture, or any other specific social location where we as humans experience the world. Autoethnography can shed light on what is happening in society because it discloses the vulnerability of the person who is describing his or her experience while situating that private world within the social and cultural context. It "incorporates a focus on interpreting the micro practices of everyday life and a critical questioning of the established social order" [25]. Autoethnography can therefore acknowledge the influence of power in systems—how the individual is both subject to that power and also is or may become a wielder of that power over others. As someone who chose to become a family doctor at a time when we talked about family medicine as *counter-culture* [26], I (LMC) was keenly aware of the power of my role and the need to consistently address the potential for abuse of that power. In my work, I tried to prioritize the use of that power on the patient's behalf whenever possible and worked consistently to avoid the easy abuse of that power. But my choice to retire did not take patients' needs into primary consideration. That would come later in the process. Although potentially useful, we could find no autoethnographic literature pertinent to this review.

Can Retirement Be an Act of Resistance?

My (LMC) decision to retire when I did I now consider to be an act of resistance. To take care of myself and to make clear my objection to the structure of my work, I needed to leave it. It was no longer possible to practice medicine the way that I felt was morally acceptable in the system in which I found myself. I had already been suffering from *disenfranchised grief*. Lathrop [27] describes multiple forms of workplace transitions in medicine that can cause physician burnout and losses resulting in grief. When the buildup of such losses in the work experience undermines the integrity of the person, the worker experiences a "mourning of the loss of a part of oneself engaged in work" [28, 29].

These words rang true to me when I thought about how the details of the practice of caring for patients in the health center where I had worked for 42 years had changed in the preceding few years. I am referring here to the increasing invasion of clinical work by the electronic medical record (EMR) with its requirements to engage with the computer during the medical encounter rather than take care of the patient. This clerical and administratively driven "work" within the computerized medical record was overwhelmingly driven by the demands of billing systems rather than the need to document the patient's narrative, medical history, physical exam, or other relevant concerns, such as social and family context. In short, the patient got lost within the attention to the machine.

References

1. Silver MP, Hamilton AD, Biswas A, Warrick NI. A systematic review of physician retirement planning. Hum Resour Health. 2016;14(1):67.
2. DeWitt TG, Roberts KB. Teaching residents about patient and practice termination in community-based continuity settings. Arch Pediatr Adolesc Med. 1995;149(12):1367–70.

3. Serwint J, Johnson P. When patients and pediatricians say good-bye in a pediatric resident continuity clinic. Arch Pediatr Adolesc Med. 1995;149(7):812–6.
4. Onyura B, Leslie K. In reply to Auster. Acad Med. 2016;91(3):289–90.
5. Onyura BP, Bohnen JMD, Wasylenki DMD, Jarvis AMD, Giblon BMD, Hyland RMD, et al. Reimagining the self at late-career transitions: how identity threat influences academic physicians' retirement considerations. Acad Med. 2015;90(6):794–801.
6. Kalet AL, Fletcher KE, Ferdman DJ, Bickell NA. Defining, navigating, and negotiating success: the experiences of mid-career Robert wood Johnson clinical scholar women. J Gen Intern Med. 2006;21(9):920–5.
7. Silver MP, Pang NC, Williams SA. "Why give up something that works so well?": retirement expectations among academic physicians. Educ Gerontol. 2015;41(5):333–47.
8. Silver MP, Williams SA. Reluctance to retire: a qualitative study on work identity, intergenerational conflict, and retirement in academic medicine. Gerontologist. 2016;58(2):320–30.
9. Curtis P. The older I get, the better I used to be. Fam Med. 2000;32(8):573–4.
10. Macaulay AC. Saying good-bye: termination of the doctor-patient relationship. Fam Med. 1992;24(1):64–5.
11. Hergott LJ. Aspects of ending a lifelong dream. JAMA. 2017;317(2):137–8.
12. Justin R. Retire and practice. Perm J. 2002;6(3):57–8.
13. Boekelheide PD. Termination and transfer of patients in family practice. J Fam Pract. 1978;6(5):1019–24.
14. Loxterkamp D. Doctors' work: eulogy for my vocation. Ann Fam Med. 2009;7(3):267–8.
15. Merenstein B, Merenstein JH. Patient reflections: saying good-bye to a retiring family doctor. J Am Board Fam Med. 2008;21(5):461–5.
16. Shorer Y, Biderman A, Levy A, Rabin S, Karni A, Maoz B, et al. Family physicians leaving their clinic—the Balint group as an opportunity to say good-bye. Ann Fam Med. 2011;9(6):549–51.
17. Brill A, Lockshin MD. Dancing at the river's edge: a patient and her doctor negotiate life with chronic illness. Tucson, AZ: Schaffner Press; 2009.
18. Penque S, Snyder M. Presence [webpage]. https://nursekey.com/presence/.
19. Pinsky E. Mortal gifts: a two-part essay on the therapist's mortality. Part I: untimely loss. J Am Acad Psychoanal Dyn Psychiatry. 2002;30(2):173–204; discussion 5–10.
20. Feller A. Termination. Panel report. J Am Psychoanal Assoc. 2009;57(5):1185–95.
21. Viorst J. Experiences of loss at the end of analysis: the analyst's response to termination. Psychoanal Inq. 1982;2(3):399–418.
22. Balint M. On the termination of analysis. Int J Psychoanal. 1950;30:184–90.
23. Ramondetta LM, Sills DR. The light within: the extraordinary friendship of a doctor and patient brought together by cancer. New York, NY: William Morrow; 2008.
24. Frank AW. Philoctetes and the good companion story. Enthymema. 2016;14:119–27.
25. Mischenko J. Exhausting management work: conflicting identities. J Health Organ Manag. 2005;19(3):204–18.
26. Stephens GG. Family medicine as counterculture. Fam Med. 1989;21(2):103–9.
27. Lathrop D. Disenfranchised grief and physician burnout. Ann Fam Med. 2017;15(4):375–7.
28. Doka K, editor. Disenfranchised grief: recognizing hidden sorrow. New York, NY: Lexington Books; 1989.
29. Trudel L, Vonarx N, Simard C, Freeman A, Vézina M, Brisson C, et al. The adverse effects of psychological constraints at work: a participatory study to orient prevention to mitigate psychological distress. Work. 2009;34(3):345–57.

Chapter 8
Facing Retirement: Grieving the Loss of Clinical Relationships

Lucy M. Candib and Eydie I. Kasendorf

Editors' Introduction

This essay intentionally follows the literature review (see Chap. 7), where we discovered the rarity of physicians acknowledging and revealing their vulnerability and emotions when discussing leaving relationships. Not anymore! Co-written by a psychologist and a family doctor about the process of ending some 200 relationships, what follows opens the entry to their and our hearts. Beyond the parallels with termination in psychiatric treatment, the joint process of paying attention to and writing about retirement becomes a way of documenting for others a person's self-reflection that situates the experience in a broader social and political context. It is a dialogic reflection that allows the exploration of personal vulnerability for the purpose of revealing the broader dynamics at work in a family, an organization, a culture, or any other specific social location where we as humans experience the world. The title tells the tale. Emotion ("grieving"), tragedy ("loss"), "relationships," and intimacy ("facing") all merge at a critical bittersweet life cycle moment ("retirement").

Expect nothing less from Lucy Candib. Although a peer and a colleague, she has served as a guide and visionary force for so many of us. She helped define feminism within family medicine and persistently served as a powerful voice for the vulnerable throughout her career. For more than 40 years, Lucy has been immersed in relationships with vulnerable families and individuals suffering from abuses of power and inequity. She's witnessed terrible loss and stunning resilience. She's taught, coached, shared, sacrificed, given, protected, persisted, struggled, and helped co-create change, and all of it filled her with meaning. She found deep love

---

L. M. Candib (✉) · E. I. Kasendorf
Department of Family Medicine and Community Health, University of Massachusetts Chan Medical School, Worcester, MA, USA

© The Author(s), under exclusive license to Springer Nature Switzerland AG 2023
L. M. Candib, W. L. Miller (eds.), *Family Doctors Say Goodbye*, https://doi.org/10.1007/978-3-031-33654-6_8

and purpose in living in those heart-cracking, heart-opening relationships. And now—retirement! Imagine the meanings being threatened. What's being lost? She is pushed to remember who she's been and how to preserve that integrity as she faces the decision to end it. How come she left her dream job?

Fortunately for her, at age 70, she was already past the average age when most women physicians retire. She did not need to feel she was retiring "early," although previously she had never seriously considered retirement. Rather, she needed to find a way to process that decision for herself and her patients, hence her work with Eydie. Their decision to document this process for others contributes to the literature about individuals struggling in a dysfunctional system and, more specifically, the processes the physician must both experience and respond to as a coherent way to withdraw from professional work while caring for herself and for her patients. Also, so very fortunately for both, they were able to forge a friendship with each other through the process of Lucy's accepting and grieving the losses involved in retiring from the long-term practice of family medicine. Working with patients' responses to her departure provided a process of healing for her long-shouldered burden of loss. Thus, Lucy's grief and loss evolved from a disenfranchised form to a clear and chosen acceptance of the need for change—for herself. Both emerged with new understandings of themselves and their life work as well as their work together. Read and be changed.

Introduction

I must admit that part of me was actively looking forward to retirement and freedom from the worsening constraints of the electronic medical record (EMR). In the previous few years, the EMR had taken over my time at home and left me no time to do the writing that I wanted to pursue. Previously, I don't think I had ever seriously considered retirement. I had worked 3 days a week for many years, but the EMR and the insistent 24-7 presence of its clinical demands when I was not in the office increasingly robbed me of my days off and my evenings to address issues that used to wait for the next day. Anyone anywhere in the health center could send me a "task" that needed action, unfiltered by any nurse or colleague, at any time. Anyone anywhere in a large hospital system could send me an email about a patient of mine at any time, sometimes with very urgent issues. There was no respite. Not to mention the demands of documentation in the poorly functioning EMR itself. Suffice it to say that after every clinical session, I would find myself in the evening sitting in front of my computer, gritting my teeth, saying, "I hate it, I hate it, I hate it," as I spent 3–4 h in documenting the work I had done that day. I recognized the life contradiction of repeating these words as I was doing what had become the "work" of my cherished and chosen profession. Not the way I wanted to be in the world. Not the way I wanted to work. Not the same profession I had devoted my life to. Thus, perhaps a few years before I would have chosen to stop seeing patients, my clinical career was brought to a close by the irrational and time-wasting effect of the intrusion/incursion of the electronic medical record (EMR) into my daily life. I made the decision to retire when I had never thought I would.

This essay, written by a family doctor with help from a consulting psychologist, is an exploration of the process of ending some 200 relationships in the months leading up to my retirement. My decision to document this process for others, with Eydie's help, was my attempt to show the doctor struggling in a dysfunctional system, documenting my own and a therapist's observations, and, more specifically, the processes that the physician must both experience and respond to as a coherent way to withdraw from professional work while caring for herself and for her patients. My work with Eydie fostered the process of my accepting and grieving the losses involved in retiring from the long-term practice of family medicine.

As someone who had chosen to become a family doctor at a time when we talked about family medicine as a counterculture [1], I was keenly aware of the power of my role and the need to consistently address the potential for abuse of that power. In my work, I tried to prioritize the use of that power on the patient's behalf whenever possible and work consistently to avoid the easy abuse of that power. But my choice to retire did not take patients' needs into primary consideration. That would come later in the process. My decision to retire at the time that I did was an act of resistance.

To take care of myself and to make clear my objection to the structure of my work, I needed to leave it. It was no longer possible to practice medicine the way that I felt was morally acceptable in the system in which I found myself. I had already been suffering from what Lathrop [2], citing the work of Kenneth Doka [3], calls *disenfranchised grief*. Lathrop describes multiple forms of workplace transitions in medicine that can cause physician burnout and losses resulting in grief. She cites Trudel et al. that when the buildup of such losses in the work experience undermines the integrity of a person, the worker experiences a "mourning of the loss of a part of oneself engaged in work [4]." These words rang true to me when I thought about how the details of the practice of care of patients in the health center where I had worked for 42 years had changed in the preceding few years.

Stories

One aspect of many years in practice is the collection of stories and mental images that have accumulated in my brain and sometimes as documents and photos over the decades. The original stories are long gone, paper records relegated to one after another storage company as folders got bigger. We used to have family folders, where each member of the family would have a folder within the larger external folder, with numbers like -01, -02, -03 for each family member. When the medical records department prepared to purge a lot of pages from especially fat folders, I would always try to save the paper record of my first visit with the patient so that we could look back on it. I also saved the genogram I had constructed on many families that I would review during "annual" visits, asking in a global way, "Any changes here?" referring to the diagram we had created. All gone. All gone with the advent of electronic medical records.

Only the stories remain, imperfectly, in fragments, only in my head, and of course, in the lived experience of the patients. But even those still seen at the health center now don't have the four-generation memories I have of their grandparents' illnesses and preoccupations. The older woman with severe rheumatoid arthritis in the late 1970s who developed a terrible vascular disease that ultimately killed her; her daughter who was the only person I ever recommended for sterilization before age 21 because of her nine pregnancies (three kids, three abortions, three miscarriages); her daughter with migraines and four biracial kids; the oldest who got in trouble, cleaned up, came home, and started a family. What a story! And from many, the photos—of newborns or of families at Christmas, which I kept in photo albums and envelopes in desk drawers. The medical records spanning the generations became the "vessels" that carried the memories, and I became the "keeper of the records." One retiring HIV specialist captured this sentiment: "(T)he memories of my patients' decades of life with a dire disease will become theirs alone. Their old paper medical records are off in storage now, and their digital charts are full of inane computer-speak, cut and pasted into gibberish [5]."

With the demise of paper, all that was left were my memories and the photos I had kept over the years. One event encapsulated the meaning of my role. This interaction happened a few months before I retired. Some of the details have been revised to make the family unrecognizable; I have the family's permission to publish it in this form.

> Teresa's mother, Tammy, had been my patient since her first pregnancy; she had three boys and two girls. Life was hard. Her first son got killed at age 8 while crossing a busy street. She never got over it. One of her partners had AIDS, and she worried about that. She did get Hep C. The boys grew up, and predictably, trouble was never far away. One son was in jail for seven years and got out, cleaned up, and was on the straight and narrow until one night, while he was on his own street, someone put a bullet through his head. Another son OD'ed. One of her sisters, LeeAnn, was also my patient. She liked her cigarettes and alcohol. She moved to California, met Mr. Right, and lived happily ever after until Mr. Right died, and she came back to town. She and Tammy just drank and drank. LeeAnn had a bunch of benzos and talked about killing herself. Tammy took them away from her, but one night, LeeAnn begged her for some and said she wouldn't do anything. Tammy gave in. But the next morning, LeeAnn was dead in her bed. LeeAnn's two children were also my patients; Tara OD'ed in her late teens. I last saw Kendrick at Tammy's funeral, and it was clear he had been using. He looked like shit.
>
> In all this, I took care of Teresa, the older of Tammy's two girls. She had a regular job in an insurance office and was raising her son. She got a new boyfriend, and it was working well, and they had a baby together. Meanwhile, Tammy was drinking steadily, lost in the guilt and grief over LeeAnn's death. She was getting worse and worse from her cirrhosis and ultimately ended up in a coma on a vent. She was shipped from the hospital to a rehab, where Teresa said the care was awful, and two weeks later Tammy was back at the hospital with a fever and aspiration pneumonia. She died when Teresa was five months pregnant. The funeral brought back all the family funerals I had attended. It took weeks to bury her because the gravesite was under the name of Teresa's older brother, who happened to be in the state penitentiary. He had to sign a paper to allow his mother to be buried at the designated site, and the paperwork was endless. Finally, she was buried.

I made it to Teresa's delivery, a sweet baby girl. Tears and joy over a baby who would never see her grandmother. Tammy was right there in the room with us in spirit after the delivery. Teresa and I were both crying. 8 weeks postpartum, I put in a Nexplanon, but she had gotten pregnant the week before, so I had to take it out the next week. So, another pregnancy. When I saw her daughter in the stroller at the prenatal visits, I kept noticing how much she looked like all of Teresa's older brothers when they were babies. I remembered how they looked. I was telling her that, and she said,

"We have no pictures. All the kids' baby pictures burned up in a fire."
"I have pictures," I said.
"You do????"

I walked out of the exam room to my office and took a photo album off a shelf. Tammy had sent me a baby picture of every single one of her babies. And some later photos too. I brought the album to Teresa, and we pulled out all the brothers' pictures. Toward the last few pages, she squealed, "That's ME!" I had her picture and one of her sister's, Darling, too.

"They're yours," I said. "I don't need them anymore."

We were both crying, for different reasons. She because of recapturing something thought lost forever, me because I could make this connection across the decades between her and her mother, both as young mothers with newborns. And because I could give her this tangible evidence of the love her own mother had been able to give her infants before the chaos. I cried also because her mother, whom I had loved through many hard times, was gone from her daughter's life, and I was going to be gone from her life soon too. That one moment exemplified my life work in family medicine that I would soon be bringing to a close.

Lucy: Background

Understanding the meaning of retirement for me requires looking back at what I thought I was doing as a family doctor over the years. Let me say, first, that I was clear from the beginning of my career that I wanted to practice in one place for my whole life as a family doctor. Secondly, I was committed to practicing at a community health center, where I could continue my political commitment to working-class and low-income families and families of color, as well as immigrant families in an urban setting. As an activist in the anti-war movement during college and medical school, I was well aware of the large external forces that robbed these families of power over their lives—the draft, the limited educational opportunities, the low-paying jobs, essentially segregated housing, and so on. Health care was another arena where power belonged to those in charge and not to patients. I was committed to leveling that power differential in my work.

Third, as a feminist and early participant in the women's health movement, I was deeply committed to the care of women and children and, after a few years, to providing full-spectrum maternity care while practicing in the health center setting. With time and with the advance of the women's movement, the rape crisis movement, and the rising awareness of violence against women, it became increasingly clear to me that many of the physical and emotional symptoms and indeed illnesses that patients suffered originated in the humiliation, neglect, and physical and sexual abuse that they had experienced as children, adolescents, and often for women, as adults. Here again, lack of power was central to their experiences. I believe I was one of a group of pioneers who tried to educate medicine about the devastating impact of such experiences on people's later health, particularly but not only for women. I remember how hard it was to convince family medicine educators in the 1980s and 1990s—when there were far fewer women family physicians and when only a handful of people would come to my talks about incest and sexual abuse—how much harm against women and children went unrecognized by their physicians.

Some ancient history about my origins in family medicine may clarify. I read Michael Balint's seminal book, *The Doctor, His Patient, and the Illness,* for the first time after my internship while I was seeing outpatients at the White River Junction VA Hospital before entering a family medicine residency. I knew that I had connected with a voice that put relationships and their maintenance at the center of patient care but also in the care of the doctor herself—despite the *His* in the title of his book. On the day I interviewed for a second-year residency slot in a just-starting residency, I discovered that John Frey, at that moment the first residency director of the program I chose, who later became my good friend, had also been reading Balint. We spent most of the interview time and another hour afterward talking about what the book meant for family medicine.

Balint and Balint groups made sense to me: relationships are central to patient care, and the doctor's own history of relationships affects how s/he could relate to patients and their problems. I realized, as all of us in that first Balint group did, that I could think better about patient-care relationships if I understood my own history intersecting with that of the patient. At the same time, I recognized that nothing related to Balint groups was remotely feminist—a concept foreign to my fellow Balint group members back in 1975. Still, my own emerging feminism mandated that relationships with patients be made more horizontal, that I learn to renounce the authoritarian prerogative of male medicine and of Balint and *his* groups of male GPs.

Of course, being egalitarian is all well and good, but I was aware that my own privilege—white, educated, professional, economically stable—meant that I almost always had more power in relationships than did my patients. Another aspect of that power came from the need and expectation of authority that patients wanted from a doctor—even as I was trying to dismantle that power itself. As with teachers, the doctor becomes a stand-in for the parent, like it or not. Patients who had had unhappy, destructive, or abusive relationships with parents or other authorities were likely to have difficult relationships with medical authorities, however kindly and egalitarian. I came to understand the dynamics of transference as one of the driving forces in the relational aspect of my work of doctoring. Consequently, I understood that the ending of clinical relationships invokes all the power of the transference that emerges from the patient's past—not to mention the doctor's countertransference issues—in other words, my own.

Putting all this in a non-technical way, I would say that over the years, with incremental understanding, I came to recognize how, for some patients, a long-standing clinical relationship with a non-abusive, caring clinician could promote healing of earlier wounds from authority figures. I believe that such a relationship fostered the potential for patients to recover their health as they came to recognize—and later move on from—the damaging effects of their early experiences in families, with parents and with partners, on their psychological and physical health. Staying loyal to and consistent with my patients as they matured and gained insight into their lives enabled me to demonstrate a kind of caring that was different from what they had experienced in the past. Some were able to shape their own parenting in a different way from what they had experienced as I followed them through their own childbearing and childrearing. I hoped that these patients would be able, ultimately, to manage the emotional loss of my retirement.

But, you might say, transference and countertransference are dynamics from psychoanalysis, and you were practicing medicine, not seeing patients twice a week in therapy for years and years. That statement is true; I was doing different work. However, the impact of decades of doing family doctoring with the same individuals and families, of being the same steady person, of being a stabilizing, consistent, caring figure in their lives, created the kind of strong relationship that generates transference in those who receive it.

As for countertransference, from my earliest beginnings as a clinician, I was always interested in the subject of *termination*—a term with psychoanalytic origins but used more loosely in therapeutic situations to refer to the process of ending clinical relationships. My interest likely stems from the tenuous and lost relationships I experienced as a child—losses that shaped the person I am, and losses I have tried to reshape over the years into positive strengths. I have written about the disappearance of my father from my life when I was small, his addiction, my parents' separation, and when I was 10 years old, his death from a stroke at age 57. Added to this was my mother's own inability to be affectionate toward a child while she herself was dealing with an addicted husband, suffering her own losses, and trying to function as a single mother and keep up appearances [6]. An additional loss for me as a young adult occurred when my first serious boyfriend was killed in Zimbabwe, where a truck collided with the tractor he was driving. I had no opportunity to grieve his death, as I was at that moment on my psychiatry rotation in my third year of medical school. With this personal history of reverberating losses, I have always been aware of the underlying needs—often unspoken and sometimes unconscious—that patients bring to the doctor-patient relationship. Because of my needs and theirs, I knew from early on that I would have to look out both for myself *and* my patients as I conducted my part of the connection between us. And, as will become clear, this recognition clarified the work I needed to do with patients and for myself in order to retire.

When facing the process of retirement, as something I had never done before, I "wanted to do it right," whatever that might be. I knew that part of it was going to be a grieving process for me and for my patients. I worried for them that "I wouldn't do it right," partly because I knew that my own issues with loss could get in the way of my "doing it right," whatever that would mean. It wasn't that I thought I *couldn't do* it. If there is someone who will put her head down and keep trudging through the hard places, I am that person. But I didn't want to do it *badly.* And "badly" would mean "not dealing with the feelings."

Doing it "Right"

It had been 30 years since I had been in therapy, but at this point I recognized that I was going to need help again. One likely reason why I had stayed in one place for so long (42 years) was that I could not imagine the idea of the losses (of relationships) that would have been involved in leaving for another job. I knew retirement would involve a grieving process, and I knew that grieving was very hard for me. With this projected sadness in mind, I wanted someone to accompany me, keep me on a steady course, provide a shoulder to lean on when it got rough, and push me when I was shutting down on the patients' feelings (typical for me to shut down if I don't want to handle or feel that I can't handle the feelings of the moment). I knew that therapy could give me a bit of distance to process the feelings and allow me some perspective. And I knew it could help me help my patients through it. So, I called Eydie Kasendorf and left a message on her machine that I wanted help with termination with the several hundred adult patients that I would be leaving. I wanted to be "the same kind of saying-goodbye-doctor that I had been taking-care-of-doctor"—something Eydie captured me saying early on in the process of working on retirement.

I chose Eydie because I wanted someone who knew about family medicine, who knew what kinds of deep attachments family doctors make with patients, and also someone who knew about the relationship dynamics of transference and countertransference that would be a part of leaving such a long-term practice. I knew that Eydie was an experienced Balint group leader, although we had never worked in the same group together. Eydie had, however, been a scribe for the faculty Balint group I had helped start when she was a graduate student and I was a young attending physician, so we were familiar with each other but had no active social or professional relationship. At the same time, I started to read about termination because I wanted to see how the closure of relationships was understood by those who practiced it deliberately: analysts whose role it is to think about how and when to end relationships. I wanted to know how to do it "right," and I wanted to know how it affected them.

I was also aware that I was about to undergo an enormous alteration in my identity. I had always wanted to be a doctor and could not imagine being anything else (when I was three years old and my father was still in practice, I picked up the phone at home and answered, "Dr. Candib's office.") Stopping practicing also meant "losing the father in me." Another way I thought about it was as taking off a very heavy coat with the pockets all filled with important tools and references and books, akin to the intern's jacket I had worn so proudly. I knew I would feel relieved by removing the heavy mantle, but I might feel insignificant or empty, like a non-entity, without the familiar but oppressive weight.

The Therapist's Perspective: Eydie

Written by Eydie Kasendorf, Ph.D.

I spent some time between Lucy's initial phone call and the first meeting in January thinking about what kind of relationship and the nature of the work that this process with Lucy would be. Because of the different boundaries and ethical considerations in the relationships between psychologists and their clients/patients, it was very important to me to give this adequate thought *before* starting.

Lucy and I were not friends or co-workers, so there was no professional boundary issue regarding dual relationships. We were "loosely related" through Family Medicine, by working with the same trainees but never had any regular professional or personal contact. I also worked half-time in the Outpatient Psychiatry Department and the Family Medicine Department as a Balint group leader. I have a long-term private practice. I was going to see her through my professional practice, and not in the department's clinical offices, which were actually located in the same building in which Lucy worked! This convenient arrangement was both for her privacy, as well as leaving open the possibility that this work could evolve into a longer-term professional relationship if needed. She was not a patient with a diagnosis (at least not initially), so it was not appropriate to bill her health insurance. She wanted to pay for my services. I consulted with colleagues about reasonable fees for this type of consultation and the appropriateness of working together (regarding any attention to boundaries). They said they did not see any professional boundary violations and suggested what the reasonable/customary fees are for this type of consultation. I contacted Lucy and we began this part of her professional journey. It was not clear at the outset what this relationship would look like (a combination of coaching and treatment), so it was crucial to discuss this at the outset and for both of us to continue to evaluate this throughout the process of our work together.

Through my work in the residency program, I knew enough about Lucy to know that she was fiercely strong and passionate about the work and seemed to many to have a "larger than life" presence. I was immediately sensitive to the possibility that working with her while she was in a more vulnerable state was something that could be uncomfortable for both of us if not addressed with both delicacy and strength.

Lucy explained in the first phone contact that she was looking to meet with me professionally as part of my work "as a psychologist and therapist" and "as someone who understood what it meant to be a family doctor" (less explaining was necessary for her). But honestly, one of my thoughts was, "How can she actually do this?" I knew enough about her relational doctoring to know that she and her patients were deeply intertwined. I wondered, "How does one divorce so many people simultaneously?" Immediately, I knew that the task of caring/helping the patients through this, and the doc, was going to be the goal.

Lucy and I met and discussed the overall plan, including the practical and psychological issues, logistics of the schedule, meeting places, fee, and the consultation/therapist role. She hired me for the job!

And so we began:

Our first meeting on January 5, 2016 was mostly an overview. We discussed Lucy's reasons for retiring: the increase in administrative/computer time (which she loathed) that was negatively affecting patient contact time (which she loved). She wanted to stop clinical care because she "had little time to do anything else." She wanted to plan the termination and not have a precipitous departure (e.g., for health reasons). This decision was also related to having a significantly older life partner. She wanted healthy time with him while they both still had it.

I asked her what her retirement would look like in a year, what types of activities, and what types of contact. It was important for me to understand her expectations at that time. Given that she was leaving between 200 and 400 patients, I did know enough about her to know that these were multi-generational, multi-stage, lifelong relationships, and that she was also a teacher/mentor. I wanted to know "how hard the stop would be." How much contact with patients, colleagues, and residents would there still be? She was hoping to continue some precepting about twice a month. She would interact with patients as part of that, but not clinically as their doctor. She would go to wakes and funerals if she knew about them. She might consider email, but no phone calls, no home visits. We talked about her personal tasks ahead (how to prepare for the gigantic changes in her life) and the institutional ones (how/when to tell patients, picking new doctors for them, for example).

She had already made a number of decisions about this process. She was going to be 70 that coming May and was planning to throw a big birthday/retirement party, inviting all of her patients and staff at the health center. I admit I was a bit shocked about this. This was the first big example of the differences in boundaries between physicians and psychologists and their patients. HIPAA popped into my head immediately, but I quickly realized that patients often have contact with each other, in waiting rooms, or even attending funerals of their beloved doctors. She wasn't planning to introduce them to each other; each person would be invited as an individual or family with a relationship to Lucy. And given the multi-generational relationships that spanned many births, deaths, and other notable occasions, for *this* doctor, with *these* patients, it made sense, and it fit. She also wanted to give patients something tangible and had already begun working on a goodbye bookmark with a picture and a message in multiple languages to give them. She was thinking about the "last" appointments a few months ahead, which she called "Taking Stock" appointments in which she and the patients could "make meaning" of their history together and the work that had been done over time. She wanted to take pictures together for a memory book, if practically possible. (It did not turn out to be feasible in the course of her clinical sessions to make this idea happen.)

I asked her what would be most hard about this for her. She was very sensitive to the fact that this *would* be very hard on her as well as on the patients. This would be a lot of loss at once, which was daunting. She had never done THIS before and was meeting with me so that she could do THIS right, as she had done so many other new things throughout her career. It was clear that the nature of our work with patients was quite similar, despite coming from different professions. She said, "I want to be the same kind of saying-goodbye doctor that I was taking-care-of-doctor." I was hooked.

In our next meeting, the work continued in a fashion that has been "the nuts and bolts" of both Lucy's and my work with patients. I constructed her four-generation genogram. To help identify what potential areas of difficulty might lay ahead for Lucy, it was important for me to get a broader understanding of her personal development, family-of-origin issues, history of attachments and losses, as well as a theory of why she became a doctor and what it meant to her in the context of her family history. Professional identities are, of course, a major part of self-concept and social roles in general, but understanding the personal significance for Lucy was a critical step in navigating this journey.

I read Lucy's book, *Medicine and the Family*, to further understand the professional significance and relational perspective of her work and noted the importance of keeping attention on the intimacy and power issues in this termination process. We also discussed her nuclear family and the history and course of her adult relationships and losses. The profound importance of the acknowledgment and validation of the *relationship* in *relational* work would be another understanding that would inform our task. This was an important part of the process for me in terms of constructing and abiding by the complex goals ahead. The narrower (and more person-centered) goal was to help Lucy deal with the impact of the loss and change involved in a transition as profound as retirement. The larger (and more relational) goal was to make sure that she continued to be true to her own core values in terms of focusing on "the other" and the relationship. My job was to help her navigate this pendulum, making sure that *she* was getting what she needed as she went through this transition and that the patients were as well. Loss and power were the key themes guiding this parallel process.

Another part was helping her manage the countertransference issues, something that she and I had both spent a lot of time on in our careers. And we both shared the Balint perspective on the importance of this, she as a long-term attendee in a faculty group and I as a long-term co-leader of resident groups. We discussed the literature we had already started reviewing before our first meeting (she, the psychoanalytic literature on termination, and me, the family medicine literature on retirement). Each of us realized that there wasn't really anything similar to what we were beginning to do together. With very few exceptions, neither literature even approached, much less addressed, the impact on the clinician. The family medicine literature covered the topic mostly with "how-to primers" for impact on patients or how to have adequate funds and hobbies post-retirement.

When I look back at our work together (meeting about every 2–3 weeks, over about 8 months), it is roughly characterized by three phases: How the EMR Ended My Career (decisions and quality of life/work issues that forced the decision to retire); Who's the Patient Here, Anyway? (the "parallel process of "taking care of Lucy" and "taking care of the patients," through Lucy, at the same time); and Life in the (Not So) Slow Lane (what the process of getting to retirement was like, and later what retired life actually looks/feels like).

For most of the time we worked together, the co-process was actually more unidirectional (with me in more of a therapist/coach role, focusing mostly on Lucy and minimizing self-disclosure), in case it needed to turn to more traditional psychotherapy, for example, if she, in fact, became depressed and needed to continue the professional sessions after retirement.

Since we were dealing with loss and change in every meeting (both current and historical), I kept an emotional and psychological "barometer" of how she was doing. Simply put, dealing with the significant and painful experiences and reactions "along the way" allowed her to proceed toward the end goal much less emotionally unencumbered than if these issues had not been addressed along the way. I was also not worried that they would surface and she would "crash" later. Our process in general was organic, and somewhat open-ended in that we continued to assess and create it as we went along. But overall, in my role as therapist/coach, I always held her psychological well-being as the primary goal. It became clear toward the end of the regular meetings together, as the retirement date approached and passed, that Lucy was emerging feeling better, lighter, more enthusiastic, and optimistic about the future, and that needing me in a more clinical role (as her therapist) was not going to be necessary.

The meetings over that period of time covered a variety of psychological and practical issues (for example, her emotional state and the emotional states of her patients, administrative tasks, and moving her things). We discussed her sadness, fears, and anxieties, as well as the mountain of work that needed to be completed before leaving. She roamed around rather freely among these topics but engaged strongly when she talked about the responses of patients when she told them she was leaving and how painful it was to "be doing this to them." She struggled with the "anxiety of destabilizing the people for whom I have been an anchor" and feeling like she was causing harm, something I very much identify with as I think about my own future work/relationship endings. At that time, I would say, "This is why I can never retire!" Somewhat coincidentally, as we were working on this paper at a much later point, after Lucy was well into her retirement, I had to take a medical leave of absence for a total knee replacement, with the second one scheduled 6 months later. The impact on so many patients for whom I am an anchor has been tricky to navigate, especially when in a "compromised" state myself. I thought about how Lucy had managed it.

In our meetings, Lucy shared the reactions of her patients to her news of leaving and their impact on her. For example, "But you're the only doctor I've ever seen!" "What am I going to do?" "The only reason I come here/put up with this place is because of you." And from a feisty 80-year-old woman, "Good for you!"

As I listened to her accounts of these interactions, I identified both with Lucy and the heaviness of "doing this" as a clinician, as well as with the patients ("having this done to them"). My own primary care doctor of 33 years had died suddenly of a heart attack. After the initial shock and acute feeling of grief and sadness, I was overcome with profound loss related to the experience that he had been present in my life for so long, through so many life stages and transitions, and that because of that, he "knew me" better than most people. I obviously survived, recovered, and found a new doctor. But that initial experience was definitely similar to losing a family member.

Because Lucy's retirement was planned, she had an opportunity to offer the patients some processing "within the context of the close relationship." This material became an essential component of the work we were doing together. In other words, what Lucy hoped to "build in" to these goodbye/last appointments was an opportunity for reflection and sharing about the doctor-patient relationship and its meaning (possibly to both of them). To be able to do this, Lucy needed an outlet/ space for processing her own feelings (being taken care of herself) so that she could continue to be present for the patients and to take care of them during this last task of their relational work together. Our meetings were a context where sadness, loss, guilt, fear, and other feelings could be managed, and Lucy could receive attention to her needs at the same time that she continued to manage the needs of her patients through this potentially painful transition. She tried to mitigate the pain—the taking stock appointments, the bookmarks, the party, hand-picking their next doctor—but that was a lot to do.

It would be necessary for Lucy to tolerate the discomfort of her experience of being the person creating the disempowerment in the doctor-patient relationships as well as tolerating the negative reactions of any patients. I knew I would have to discourage Lucy from sugar-coating or rationalizing and instead help her manage both her guilt and the potential sadness and anger coming from patients. The decision to end these hundreds of relationships was unilateral; patients had no vote, no say. This would be the first—and if not the first, certainly the biggest—example of what she had spent her career avoiding: disempowering people she cared for. It was crucial for her to be sensitive to the needs of the patients going through this and for me to be sensitive to hers. As a resident Balint Group leader for over 25 years, I was well-practiced in "taking care of docs taking care of patients." And of course, this was why she chose to work with me, particularly during this transition in her career.

Saying Goodbye Is Hard!

Some patients presented particular emotional challenges. One, whom Lucy had known for 42 years since the patient was 14, was now dying. Another was an incest survivor whom Lucy had worked with for over 25 years, had gone through a chaotic young adulthood, and finally became a gifted clinician working with disturbed adolescents. We spent many sessions working on how to best navigate these endings.

Sadness and guilt, especially, needed to be addressed in our work so that Lucy could continue to be as present (and non-defensive) as possible during these emotionally intense transitions and also be able to tolerate the reactions of the patients (which could be quite painful). I continued to assuage any guilt ("You are allowed to leave."). I believe one of the important pieces of our work together (and of this kind of endeavor, retirement, in general) is being able to discuss and work through the current sadness and experience of loss while remembering resolved or unresolved prior losses and being able to manage the flooding feelings and able to handle their impact.

Lucy: Reflection on These Losses

As Eydie points out, one of the two women who were particularly difficult to leave was one I will call Mary, who was actively dying during the first 3 months I worked with Eydie. She died 2 months before my retirement date. I was glad for the timing because I couldn't imagine trying to transfer her to another clinician while she was dying.

Mary's past was lost in the dust of social service history. Her mother had died when she was 10, and Mary became a "ward of the state," bouncing from one foster care to another. I met her when she was about 14, supposedly in some program or other, but I never could figure out what it was. She was drinking a lot, cutting, and yelling and swearing whenever she didn't get what she wanted from our health center. She worked the streets for money for cigarettes and booze. I only heard from her when she wanted something. I sewed up a fair number of self-inflicted lacerations on her forearms when things got really bad for her. Interactions consisted of her yelling, swearing, demanding, begging, and often walking out without being seen if she had to wait more than a few minutes. I refused to see her or talk on the phone with her if she was drunk. Otherwise, I just kept plugging along. About 10 years into it, she became pregnant, ironically about the same time I was pregnant with my second child, and we were even in the hospital at the same time.

She went on to have a total of four children. When the last was born, the Department of Social Services swept in and removed the newborn baby boy for permanent adoption. They also managed at that time to move all the other children to foster care, as Mary wasn't really able to look after small children. She drank, she swore at them, and she didn't supervise them. The oldest, a 7-year-old named Jessica went to one foster home, and the two middle kids, a boy and a girl, went to a different foster care together. Mary was devastated. She would get occasional communications about the older three, but the infant's adoption was anonymous. He was "somewhere in New Hampshire." Over the subsequent years, she kept smoking and drinking, did occasional cocaine when her check came in, and would bring me periodic communications from Jessica, whose foster parents would help her send an annual photo.

As time passed, her health deteriorated. She developed chronic bronchitis with a persistent cough and phlegm and chronic low back pain with gradually incapacitating degenerative joint disease in her lower spine. At age 45, she had a seriously abnormal pap smear positive for the cancer-causing HPV virus, but she refused to do anything about it. Around the same time, she also developed a cyst emerging from one labia that grew to the size of a grapefruit and came to obstruct her vaginal opening to the point that a speculum exam was not possible. I tried making her appointments with the kindest ob-gyn in town for removal of the cyst under general anesthesia to be followed by colposcopy and a biopsy of her abnormal cervix, but she refused it all. She was sure she would die under anesthesia.

Eventually, Mary came to rely on a motorized scooter as walking was too painful, and she entered into our chronic pain program so I could provide her with some opioid pain relief while under supervision. I saw her every couple months over the last 10 years for her various chronic problems, but I could never budge her about getting her cervix looked at. She used the emergency room when she had severe respiratory or abdominal complaints, always refusing hospitalization, but mostly saw me during office hours. While most public housing in our city is in the inner city or in commercial areas, one small section of public housing was located near my own home, on the more middle-class edge of town. I knew that Mary lived there from the address, but I carefully did not start making home visits, as I knew she would come to expect me to come to her rather than her getting out of the house.

About 2 years before my retirement, she began to complain of lower abdominal pain, but a CT scan of her abdomen was unrevealing except for something vague in or near her ovary. She became homebound with visiting nurses administering her opiates twice a day from a "lock-box." In the last year, she began to have intermittent heavy vaginal bleeding (still refusing evaluation) and then signs of upper GI (gastrointestinal) obstruction with vomiting of all solids, requiring an ER visit. I was finally able to get her a CT scan of her abdomen and pelvis through the emergency room, but she didn't stay over to wait for the results or any treatment.

I wrote the following about the results of the CT scan:

> *I went to her little smoke-filled apartment after work on the day the radiologist called with her CT scan report: nodules everywhere. Vomiting liquids, 30 lb. weight loss, early satiety.*
> *"I came to tell you what your CT scan showed."*
> *I asked her what she thought might be her diagnosis, and she asked,*
> *"It's bad, isn't it?" And I said,*
> *"Yes, it's spread all around."*
> *"So, what is it, anyway?"*
> *"What do you think?"*
> *"You tell me," getting aggravated.*
> *"It's cancer."*
> *"It's cancer?"*
> *"Yes, it's cancer."*
> *"See, I knew it. I told you I was having all that pain. Now you'll believe me."*
> *"Yes, I do believe you."*
> *"Well, I hope I have at least a couple years."*
> *This from the person who refused to have her chronic symptoms evaluated. "I'll take my chances," she used to say.*
> *What do I say now? Carcinomatosis is not a 2 year diagnosis.*
> *Now, crying, she says,*
> *"I guess I'll have to pack this place up."*
> *"People will help you."*
> *"And what about my cat, what's going to happen to him?"*
> *Pointing her index finger directly at me, she insisted, "You'll take him, won't you, secondhand smoke and all!"*
> *"Yes, I suppose I will." Overfed Tabby cuddled next to her, content. The only tenderness in her life. He comes and lets me pet him, purring.*
> *This one is going to be very hard.*
> *"Yes, I will take him."*
> *And I will take care of you before that, I think, for these weeks or months, but not those years you thought you had.*

All of a sudden, Mary was willing to do anything. I talked to my good friend in palliative care, who steered me toward a lovely oncological surgeon who reviewed the CT scan and brought it to the Tumor Board. The palliative plan was to have Mary admitted for relief of gastric obstruction (done endoscopically under anesthesia). Getting her admitted required arranging transportation from her home to the hospital on a Sunday (something I didn't know could be done) and dealing with the cat. She had no one to take him; it was true. My partner and I managed to go and feed him twice a day during her stay at the hospital. It was not a big chore. We practically passed her apartment anytime we went down our street to the nearest big intersection less than a mile away.

Meanwhile, I worried about who would take care of Mary if she lasted past my retirement date. She went home to the cat, able to eat and drink again. But before she could see the medical oncologist my friend had recommended, Mary ended up in the hospital with a pneumonia. This time we took the cat to our house. The oncologist saw her during that hospitalization and discussed with her the overall poor prognosis and the substantial side effects from cancer treatment that would make her miserable for the next few months and not necessarily change the outcome. Mary decided not to pursue treatment; instead, she chose to give up her apartment, give away all her possessions, and move into a nursing home for end-of-life care. She went directly from the hospital to the nursing home. Mary died there 11 days later, never having received any palliative care attention, despite it having been ordered. But that is another story. The cat got a new name, Norman, and settled in. That is how I came to take home a patient's cat. Despite Eydie's doubts, it seemed to make sense to me, within the 42-year context of my knowing Mary. The reality was that taking care of Mary had been a constant in my entire clinical life as a family doctor. Her cat was part of the inheritance. His presence in my life meant that Mary came to mind every day, and that was a good thing. Norman lived with us for several years, then 1 day he did not come back into the house. He likely met his end with the coyotes, who have taken many neighbors' cats as well. Sigh. He was gone too.

Eydie

Lucy was affected by Mary's death more than she thought she would be. When I questioned whether her taking the cat may have been motivated, in part, by guilt, Lucy responded simply, "There was no one else to take the cat, and she knew that I would." [Lucy: Thinking about it now, taking the cat was a way to keep taking care of Mary. It was continuity of care!]

At each session, Lucy would do a brief "check-in" of how much was left to do as she whittled away at the pile until 2 weeks *after* her actual last day of work. Over many of the sessions, we talked about what seemed like an impossible task: getting all the work completed, saying the goodbyes, and doing the medical part of the visit, fitting in so many people. She reported that "the appointments were good, the paperwork a killer," which was, in fact, a motivation for leaving the clinical practice at this time. At times, Lucy described "everything as sludge, like glue," so many goodbyes, wrap-ups, lab letters, and referrals still to be done.

Our sessions were full of talk about practical details for the upcoming party and clinical issues regarding difficult patients, along with bursts of "Will I have an identity? Who will I be anyway? Will I be anyone?" She shared her reaction when she offered to the medical director that she could continue working on physician recruitment on a consultative basis to being told, "We won't need you for that anymore." [Lucy: I was quite insulted by his dismissal of my offer. And in fact, physician recruitment took a bad nosedive on my departure, as he had no strengths in that area.] Her thoughts covered everything from "Will I still have a key to the building?" to "Will I have a self?" As the retirement date neared, she reported more crying throughout the process. But she also talked positively and optimistically about plans for after retirement, both related to work, precepting, writing, continuing to do asylum evaluations, engaging with medical students, as well as personally including taking better care of herself and having more time for activities she had not been able to "fit in."

Lucy

In recent years, physician retirement finally became a focus of academic interest in the form of a systematic review [7]. These authors looked at the timing of the choice of when physicians retire (early or delayed) and how the best institutions might enable physicians to work longer or plan more successfully. For some, retirement clearly serves as a form of identity threat [8]. I reverberated with this fear beforehand with the question, "Will I have a self?" yet it was not my main concern. And I did manage to keep my key to an office and a cubby in the clinical part of the health center! When professionals in their late career maintain a single-minded vision of what constitutes success, they may have more difficulty considering retirement as an option and in accepting the diversification that is necessary for a successful retirement. Onyura talks about the possibility of "reimagining the self" through new activities and finding another way to give through the family [9]. She notes that women in academic medicine may have a different transition to and vision of retirement. Because balance between family and career has usually been a goal and an accomplishment throughout their careers, later career choices may not be so problematic for women [10]. I found this true. I was looking forward to continuing to precept residents on a regular basis and on increasing my availability to teach and perform medical evaluations for asylum.

Eydie

As the beginning of May (her last month) approached, Lucy reported having to say no to requests for appointments, which was difficult. Finding time to see all of the patients was impossible; every clinical session was FULL until her last scheduled day. She fell more and more behind on charts, in part because these last notes had to "communicate a lot" since she would no longer be the "keeper of the memories" and the "mantle had to be passed." She was spending a lot of time finding new docs for her patients. Picking them personally was very important to her. I asked her if anyone else could do this, but she felt she needed to do it herself. She reported feeling a sense of relief when two of her "hardest patients" were assigned.

[Lucy: One with a diagnosis of multiple personality disorder who bounced among various personae during office visits, and the other a 43-year-old dialysis-dependent woman with end-stage heart disease on whom I made home visits and who has since died.]

One other clinical relationship required a lot of thought during this time. Karen was an incest survivor who had been Lucy's patient for over 25 years. Somehow Karen had not managed to make an appointment to see Lucy before her last day of work. Lucy was not willing to work an extra session to "fit her in." Lucy brought me her emails, seeking help with how to manage Karen's needs erupting just as Lucy was trying to disengage. Lucy would no longer be able to or want to be her anchor. We spent time discussing how best to handle this.

Lucy: Writing About Karen

At the beginning of April, I finished assigning all my patients to another doctor, almost all attending physicians, except for those who already had a good relationship with a nurse practitioner. I reassigned Karen to a senior male physician whom she had seen during my absence years ago. She had already been seeing a male cardiologist, so I thought this might work since she already knew my male colleague. She had been out of work for a couple of weeks with a prolonged viral illness when she received her letter of reassignment from me. She wrote back 6 weeks before the date when I would no longer be seeing patients with very strong feelings of loss and abandonment about which she was very realistic, but still stinging with the loss involved, mixed with gratitude for our long work together.

> *I know I'll never have a relationship like this one with any doctor, ever. I know I don't need it as much anymore, but it sure felt good. It sure felt good. Even though I don't see you as much, I feel safer knowing you are there if I need you. I'm at a place where I can hold you in my heart & grieve.*—Email April 15, 2016.

For a while she barraged me with emails reflecting the wide range of her emotions, peppered with questions about how I was doing and how I was handling it.

> *I'm wallowing in my grief. Well, I don't have much else to do right now but think. I'll suddenly think about not having you as my doctor anymore, never seeing you again & I burst into tears. My heart is breaking. I'm really going to miss you! I know it's selfish. I'm sure many of your patients are sad. How are you dealing with all that? You're only one person to me, but you've got so many patients. I am so, so grateful that I got to be one of them for such a good long time. Can you hold all of this grief for us? I know you can hold a lot of suffering, but it's different when you're the catalyst for it.*—Email April 16.

This is Karen at her most perceptive, knowing how being "the catalyst for it" meant that I would feel responsible for how my patients felt and how they might respond.

Besides sad, I feel anxious (I know. Me? Anxious? How odd). I'm trying to take better care of myself. I mean I have a future that I hadn't planned on. I really wanted you to be my doctor a bit longer. I supposed it would hurt whenever you chose to stop seeing patients. It never would have been a good time for me. I wish you could have seen more of the better me. Who else will be able to handle me when I get old? (A little denial that you will also get older.) I keep thinking of where I still struggle. It's just easier, safer with you. You know me & you're patient when I struggle to be in & to interpret my body. I never had to worry about not being heard. I can ask you stupid questions. Thanks to you, I have allowed other docs to touch me (I don't like it, but I can do it), but I don't trust them like I trust you. I can tolerate you knowing more about my body than I do. I can tolerate feeling afraid with you & know you'd never exploit it. I remember when you sent me a card after my first pap.... My heart just aches. I'm scared not to have you anymore. Especially when something about my body has made me feel vulnerable.—Email April 16.

Karen would ask dozens of questions in her emails to me about how I was handling my retirement, what I would do, what about my family, and so on. I sent back a brief email requesting, "One question at a time."

What happened to my fat chart? All that stuff you use to let me read, back in the day. (We've been through a lot of technology together.)

Do you remember all those letters I used to write to you? I wish I had a scrap book to look back on. This relationship has a long history. I'm able to appreciate it in more ways than I knew existed in the past. When I read your stuff & think about our relationship I think you really do what you write about.

I wish that you could tell me what our relationship means to you, I don't want to read it all in a book. It seems like it just happened. I got lucky that the things you were thinking & writing about were the areas where I needed to be seen and heard. Do you remember me when I was in my 20's? 30's? 40's? I think I started seeing you about the time I graduated from college. My memories from the years when I was PTSD-ing all over the place are blurry. Some non-existent. But I do remember you being there for me during some of the toughest times, and the tough times went on for years & years. I pissed you off a few times & you didn't ditch me. Sometimes I worry that I haven't done well enough in my life for all your efforts. I'm still trying. This trauma shit really affects us to the core of our beings. It seems like we spend a lifetime working things out, year after year. It never really completely goes away. It just lies dormant at times. Then it awakens to wreak some havoc. I have to untangle it from my core, shred it and continue. I find that it comes up a lot in my most important relationships and whenever I feel vulnerable (like when I'm sick). Thanks for working so hard so that now I can access healthcare. How am I ever going to thank you? How am I going to say goodbye?—Email, April 21.

I don't know how you kept patient 'just talking' with me for as long as you did. I understand that you gave me as much of the control as you could. You helped me figure out what I needed in order to allow myself to be examined. Eventually I was able to let other doctors know what I needed. AND because of our work together, I need much less than I once did. When you first told me you were retiring, I was sure I would quit going to doctors all together.... Now I'm beginning to feel that would be disrespectful to our years of work. Sad that I have to walk the rest of this journey without you. But if I had not met Lucy Candib I may have never taken the first step.—Email, April 30.

These brief excerpts are from the last 2 weeks of April. By the beginning of May, I was seeing patients packed into 15-min visits back-to-back, some who had scheduled "annual physicals" so they wouldn't have to go to the doctor for a long time, some who just came to talk. I was not keeping track of who had appointments and who didn't. The days were overwhelmingly draining. I was having trouble getting my notes done and let all my lab letters about results fall completely behind. At some point, I found out that Karen did not have an appointment scheduled. And I had no openings. After the much-anticipated party (at the end of my last week of seeing patients), she wrote:

> *No, we don't have an appointment scheduled. You told me that this coming week may be easier for you to fit me in. Is that no longer possible? This all happened so fast. I really want to be able to talk with you.*
>
> *I cried most of the drive home, filled with grief, but more so gratitude & the sense of being a small part of something huge & empowering & wonderful. You have always helped awaken my feminism & make me feel empowered. I read a bunch of old emails that I had sent to you, as far back as 1992. Reading them made me truly appreciate how you hung in there with me for years. They also showed me how far I have come in my healing process. They also document experiences I had forgotten. Got me wondering how you will remember me.*
>
> *PLEASE try your hardest to fit me in. I really need this.*—Email, May 30, 2016.

Over the years, Karen took responsibility for booking her own appointments. I did not pay attention to who did and did not have appointments in the last week that I had been scheduled to see patients. I wrote back:

> *I will try to find a time to talk on the phone. I am not seeing patients this week.* [I actually had finished seeing patients altogether.]
>
> *It will need to be time limited. Not our usual modality but that's what I have.*
> *I will let you know what will work for me.*
> *What days/times could you get 30 minutes?*
> *lucy.*

She was enraged, petulant, and begging.

> *After all these years & everything you've meant to me, I don't want to say goodbye to you over the phone! I didn't know the last time I saw you would be the last time—in life forever. I need a proper termination. I'm healthier than I have been in a long time, but I know that I need to say goodbye in a way that respects the relationship and what it has meant to me. I need this for my mental health. Just because I didn't come to see you as much as I used to, doesn't mean that you weren't important in my heart. I would have loved to have seen you regularly, but I figured I'd drive you crazy if I wasn't sick & I'd probably take the appointment from someone who really needed it. I know you've not wanted me to feel 'special,' but right now I need to advocate for myself. Too much history, too many horrors shared, too much trust built (and you know I can count the people I trust on one hand), I'm too attached, too grateful to say what I need to say and hear from you what I need to hear over the phone. You're one of the women who saved my life & helped to make it better. Please, isn't there something we could figure out to make this happen? Please.*
>
> *… the woman you have known since I was a kid in my 20s… who you spent years "just talking" to, who you wrote to from Ecuador, sent a congratulations card to after I got my first PAP, saw me last and listened to me till after everyone had gone home, sent me amazing articles to help me out in grad school. You put my name in one of your books…and who I was able to allow to be my doctor, to touch my body, to know my shame & love me anyway.*
>
> *How you going to commit to someone like that and think it's ok to say goodbye by phone? That's not how you operate. It isn't how you've operated, ever.*—Email, May 30, 2016.

I offered her some possible times to talk on the phone, I thought. But she thought I was offering her in-person appointments. So, when I offered her a 5 p.m. appointment on June 1, I was offering a phone appointment. When she realized I was still talking about a phone appointment, she responded,

I didn't think we were doing this by phone. We can't meet?—Email, May 31.

And I responded:

I feel bullied.
I don't want to do this. Have this conversation.
I finished seeing patients last week. I am shutting my practice down.
I NEED it to be over with everyone.
Yes, you are special.
But no, I don't want to meet.
I will talk to you on the phone for 30 minutes tomorrow.
You will survive this. Don't make it a big dramatic event.
If it is going to be like this, I will NOT want to be in email contact with you at all.
—Email, May 31, 2016.

We did ultimately have the appointed phone conversation. I think it was more like an hour, but I didn't keep track of it. At the time, I thought it went all right. She had my full attention, and I didn't have to do another damn note in the electronic medical record. I look back on how I was responding to her emails and see that all the feelings of being completely drained, empty of energy, and finished with work were driving me to try to shut down. I really couldn't hear anymore, I think. Karen was right. I wasn't the best I could have been, but I was as good as I was able to be at that moment. It seems both fitting and ironic that I couldn't come through for someone who had taught me so much about being a survivor. Fitting, because she still needed a lot, and ironic that my own need for self-protection prevented me from giving it. I also felt like I had disappointed Eydie, so I added another layer of self-blame on top of the guilt that I felt toward Karen for not being the same kind of saying-goodbye-doctor that I had been taking-care-ofdoctor. In short, I was not at my best, but it was all I had.

Now, almost 7 years later, I realize that some of my inertia in trying to finish writing this document about retirement is lodged in my feelings of guilt for not having done a better job of conducting this most difficult of relationship closures. I agreed with Karen. I should have seen her in person. But on the other hand, she had 7 weeks to book an appointment and didn't do it. So, then my booking something with her, something that would have to be in the evening or a time when I would not have been working, in the first week after stopping appointments, became an obstacle, a load I couldn't lift, a piece of food too big to swallow. It became the addition of *more* when my mind and my body were crying out for *less*, for needing to have it be done, for finishing the marathon, not for running another 100 yards. Somehow, metaphors about my mouth seem most apt. I felt like something was being forced down my throat, and I couldn't breathe, and I couldn't swallow. For me, saying *no* to Karen at that point felt necessary for my survival.

These words sound overly dramatic to me now, but I know, putting myself back to those days and paying attention to the tightening knot in my stomach as I write this, that I just couldn't do it. I realize now that I could not tolerate the intensity of her reactions toward the loss, and I suppose I feared that she would be demanding reprieve, ongoing connection, and control. I reacted to the increasing intensity of the emails by wanting it to be over; I needed to draw a line and close it out. I see my own limitations in ending the relationship with Karen more clearly now.

My work with Karen raises the importance of countertransference in ending complex medical relationships. In psychiatry, this process is called termination, the planned ending or goal of successful psychoanalytic or long-term treatment. Interestingly enough, even when psychiatrists address the challenges of termination, it is always the patient who has the complicated feelings (resistance, anger, regression, and hostility) that must be interpreted and managed. The occasional mention of countertransference (the therapist's response to the patient's words, actions, and feelings) omits explicit acknowledgment of the affective component of this work. The anger, loss, and grief in response to the loss of a caring relationship often lasting many years, though unmentioned, may still simmer underneath the professional stance [11]. These feelings are not discussed and are not viewed as appropriate for expression, either to the patient or even to colleagues.

Judith Viorst, a non-physician analyst probably best known for writing *Alexander and the Terrible, Horrible, No-good, Very Bad Day* [12], recognized the startling void in this area and interviewed 20 psychoanalysts, under the cloak of anonymity, about their personal reactions to the end of long-term treatment with their patients [13]. She reports that during the interviews each of them "made a serious effort at self-examination...and that because of the isolation of their work, they found pleasure and relief in talking about it ([13], p. 401)." These interviews confirm that most psychiatrists do experience but never overtly acknowledge deep feelings of sadness and loss with the closure of long-term clinical relationships. She found that some analysts were able to identify how they had used a patient's termination "to resolve some piece of their own unfinished business ([13], p. 417)."

As for me, I know I did a good job with many patients, reminding them of their strengths and all that they had accomplished over 20 or 30 or 40 years with me. As we hugged, I would whisper in a person's ear, "You were such a good mother," "You were such a good daughter to your mother," "You did the absolute best you could," and other such positive summaries of my respect for them. Like Viorst's psychiatrists describing their responses to the ending of long-term clinical relationships, I found that working with these patients' responses to my departure provided a process of healing for my own long-shouldered burden of loss. Thus, my grief and loss evolved from the "disenfranchised" form described by Lathrop to a clear and chosen acceptance of the need for change for me. In Viorst's words: "In dealing with aspects of loss, analysts may find that they can utilize their responses for their own—as well as their patients'—further development [13]." Unfortunately, for Karen, whose survivor work had spanned more than half of my career, I was unable to do this; I couldn't keep my own feelings out of it; I couldn't set aside my needs for her. I am aware now of how angry it made me that she again wanted me to make an exception for her. But the survivor in me just couldn't come through anymore for her, or anyone else, at that time. I so needed to stop having to do it that I just said *no*. It really was time for me to retire.

In retrospect, although at the time I felt that I had failed Karen, I think now that the hard stop that I placed on our relationship may have been necessary and possibly useful for her, though this may just be a justification on my part. I think about a friend and mentor of my youth, someone who knew about my father's addiction, someone whom I admired, and who knew how much I respected him. We corresponded for years. Then I got a letter from him that blew me away. He confessed to me that he had clay feet and that he knew that I would be very upset because of my father's history of addiction, but that he felt he had to tell me. He was addicted to an opiate and was going to the hospital to withdraw from it. I know now how much it cost him to write that letter. I feel the same way about confessing, in writing, that I did not do right by Karen. I was neither the doctor she thought I was nor the one I would have wanted to be. I did what I could, and in this instance, I didn't do it well. But, just as my friend's disclosure of his addiction eventually helped me understand his life and our relationship, perhaps my challenge in ending my clinical relationship as Karen wished it revealed to her that I was just a person at the end of my rope, another survivor doing the best I could. And she could grow from that.

Eydie: Comment

Reading Lucy's words now, 7 years later, I am struck by how hard she is on herself. We discussed Lucy's struggle with Karen, interpersonally as well as intrapsychically, as it was unfolding and agreed on what were reasonable options. I agree with Lucy that she did the best that she could at the time. I also believe that the ending of the specific clinical relationship with Karen symbolically came to represent the difficult, painful, and complete hard stop to her medical practice, and Lucy felt she had no other choice. That is why Lucy made these decisions with this patient at that moment in time, and it makes complete sense that she is judging herself now, looking back, but in a much healthier, less stressed state.

Lucy

You may be wondering. Before this is published, will Karen read these words? Of course! I wouldn't and couldn't publish her emails without her permission. I imagine we will have another long email exchange. I am not looking forward to that part, but I think she will be very pleased to know that I still think about her a lot.

Eydie: Closure

Another aspect of retirement from a long career, especially in one place, is the task of "removing oneself" from the physical space—from desk to books/journals, pictures, and personal mementos from patients. What does one do with all of this? Lucy's space in the health center continued to shrink and expand at home! We talked about how difficult it was to "have to give my work away" and to remove all of her things (self) from her spaces in the health center.

With 3 weeks to go and 60 lab results letters, she was trying to make them more personal. Again, this was an example, like the last appointments, of how a relational doc continues to focus on the very last moments of the relationship. But, like Peter Curtis, it's "hard to take" doing too many at a time. Besides, now there were honors, parties, new projects, and scholarships being suggested for her life work. As she was winding down all her clinical activities, she wondered, "Will I be a happy person?" And we discussed the importance of maintaining a number of the things that she did enjoy, as well as adding new ones. As she went through the last week of work, the feelings of loss/sadness, for the actual changes after decades, became more prominent. Sadly, "I'm not going to deliver babies anymore." "Last night, my last call." "All the lasts." "That week was hard, every visit." "I can't imagine not doing what I'm doing and have it be over because it's never been over." But at the same time, "I'm looking forward to time off."

As the actual retirement date neared, there was a flood of disparate emotions and tasks. Lists were being completed and lost. All patients had their new doctor assignments, and the letters were written. Details for the party needed attention, like managing the electronic invitation responses, estimating the amount of food, confirming the site would meet the DJ's requirements, and so on. Hosting an event that included a fancy dinner for 200 people in a beautiful venue in the middle of the city with music and dancing meant both excitement but also some uncertainty!

The party **was** an exceptional event! My early concerns were unfounded. As guests entered and a long line formed, Lucy greeted each guest personally. People ended up sitting either with their own family members, or mixed in with health center staff, colleagues, or friends, a beautiful blending of all who attended. There was so much warmth and affection, some speeches, and dancing! Lucy made sure to give her patients the beautiful bookmarks that she had designed and printed for them. A colleague, who gave a speech, remarked that Lucy had said early on that she wanted to work at one place her whole career. And she **had done** that. The party really seemed like the perfect way for Lucy to share her retirement and her 70th birthday with so many of the people who had been the actual essence of her lifelong career. As Lynn Carmichael wrote, the *family* in family medicine refers to the *quality of the relationships* [14].

She was preparing to go to a world family medicine conference in Brazil, feeling overwhelmed and procrastinating, "flailing among stuff and tasks." When we met "two days into retirement," Lucy still had 2 weeks of paperwork to do. The residency graduation was coming up next, and there would be a new "Lucy Candib award," for which she would be the first recipient. We worked on to-do lists, prioritizing. She had not yet "established a rhythm" with the unscheduled time. Lucy remarked, "This really is life-changing, not just here, at home too." She felt like she was "sloughing her entire skin," as she moved more things and purged large quantities of others, like entire collections of journals. She had more time for exercising, cooking, and spending time with family where the relationship with her "stay-at-home" partner also needed some attention and negotiation. "Every aspect of this is a relationship."

When she returned to the health center for her first precepting session in July, she told me she was "feeling very light" and not sad at all. After crying through but still completing the last 30 lab/goodbye letters, she loved the new schedule with more vacation time and felt that "life was good." She had a feeling of "floating," having taken off "the jacket" with all the heavy stuff, the mantle, and passing the baton.

Before she left for Brazil 3 months later, we discussed/assessed her emotional/mental state and decided she "was on the other side." She was not depressed, nor did it appear that depression was a likely outcome. We would end the professional consultation and continue as colleagues. We agreed that we might start to work on something together (this project/paper) over time. We began our collegial meetings at that time, reviewing literature, writing some sections, and sharing our experiences of the process we had gone through together. Our contact then decreased over time as we went "back to our own lives," for the most part.

My availability then dropped off significantly as a result of two major surgeries 6 months apart and leaves of absence from my two clinical practices after each of these. Returning to work each time was an ordeal, with both the need to take care of my therapy patients (who had been covered but anxiously awaited my return) and with the extremely time-consuming addition of a rigorous physical therapy schedule for 2 months after each surgery. At the same time, the focus of the manuscript, for Lucy, evolved from the narrower subject of "the retirement process" to a more amplified reflection of her life and career, culminating in the retirement process and moving on to the next stages. At this point, the final project/paper is more reflective of Lucy's journey, with my role in a particular segment of that.

At the time of this writing, Lucy has had the time to decide on which professional and personal activities she wants to engage in and is still the busiest person I know. The "termination" of relationships is complete and appears successful. After many points, when running into patients at the health center, or in public, she would show deep affection, like seeing an old friend, without the feeling of responsibility for their care. For example, one day, sometime after the retirement, when we were meeting in a café in Worcester to work on this paper, Lucy was greeted by an Albanian couple who were former patients. As they negotiated the hugs and had a brief chit-chat with some language challenges, what stood out to me was the warmth, affection, and shared history, but also the fact that all had moved on *and were okay.*

Lucy

Through all of my 40 years of practice, I functioned as a faculty member for family medicine residents during their 3 years of training at our health center. Over time, my role as an educator became increasingly clear to me, as well as the particular elements of family medicine that I was especially privileged and prepared to teach. Here was another dimension where I had to think hard about power in relationships and where patterns of relationships in residents' own families of origin sometimes emerged in their reactions to me as another parental figure in their lives. Teaching became increasingly important to me as the years went on, and gradually I realized it was one of the aspects of medicine where I hoped to stay involved after retirement. It was one aspect of "identity bridging" that made sense, that was needed, and that I could do. A second was the continuation of my work conducting and teaching medical evaluations for persons seeking asylum in the U.S. The first maintained relationships with learners and other faculty and obliged me to "keep up" with the literature; the second, also involving teaching, addressed my commitment to spend more of my time working for justice and social change.

Three years after my retirement, I wrote that I was happy with the result. I had regularly scheduled precepting sessions, supervising residents at all levels. At these sessions, I was the "second preceptor," needed when, according to ACGME rules, more than four residents were scheduled to be seeing patients. This arrangement kept me connected with faculty colleagues and allowed relationships with learners to grow. Expanding my work with asylum seekers enabled me to expose more learners to the realities of persecution around the world for persons who oppose repressive governments, for persons fleeing unbearably violent relationships, and for persons from many countries because of their gay and lesbian sexual orientation. In addition to getting more sleep and more exercise, I felt that I was continuing to be more myself as a family doctor, albeit outside of direct clinical care, but directly in relation with learners and asylum seekers. Although the output was small, I also had more time to read, write, and think, all contributing to a greater sense of accomplishment.

Then the pandemic happened. Initially, the health center closed completely, then reorganized to address the severity of illness in the community. Clinical activity at the health center changed dramatically. Primary care evaporated, and residents were all engaged in inpatient work. Later, when outpatient precepting resumed, I was not someone necessary to be there, and it seemed unwise for me to expose myself to Covid-19 when I was not actually needed, potentially jeopardizing both my health and my spouse's. I stopped going into the health center to precept, which turned out to be a great loss to me. As the pandemic settled into normality, I was able to resume doing limited medical asylum evaluations with medical student scribes, using all the standard masking precautions. This work remains illuminating and rewarding. I have also maintained involvement through Zoom, both in the weekly faculty Balint group and in an interdisciplinary group on trauma-informed care, working with colleagues to find a way to make all the clinical work at the health center be trauma-informed. Now, at the time of putting together this book in 2022, I see myself as much more retired but still missing the relationships with learners. Eydie and I have not seen each other in several years but will be working on this chapter together before the book goes into the final stages of editing.

Eydie

Lucy and I commence our conversations as I am also reducing my clinical time due to an increase in family responsibilities— after an extremely busy increase in work during the first 2 years of the pandemic. And like Lucy at the time of her retirement, I am currently experiencing managing the complex emotions of the many people "for whom I have been an anchor" as well as my own emotions. And interestingly, though not really surprisingly, I have had many contacts from former patients who have asked to come back for "some more work." Having a 40-year practice, former patients are now wanting to do some existential therapy around the issues of aging, loss, relationships, and identity. I am doing as much as I can to help, but keeping my own needs and goals in place—the very balance that Lucy and I worked on during our time together. It has been great to connect with Lucy to complete this work, and to see her in the place she is now.

Lucy

And I hope that having helped me work through my retirement will serve Eydie well as she wrestles with the same set of difficult issues with **her** 40 years of clinical relationships!

References

1. Stephens GG. Family medicine as counterculture. Fam Med. 1989;21(2):103–9.
2. Arndt BG, Beasley JW, Watkinson MD, et al. Tethered to the EHR: primary care physician workload assessment using EHR event log data and time-motion observations. Ann Fam Med. 2017;15(5):419–26.
3. Bernard HS, Drob S. "Afterwork": a clinical-phenomenological report. Psychiatry Q. 1989;60(4):359–69.
4. Trudel L, Vonarx N, Simard C, et al. The adverse effects of psychological constraints at work: a participatory study to orient prevention to mitigate psychological distress. Work. 2009;34(3):345–57.
5. Zuger A. Moving on. N Engl J Med. 2018;378(19):1763–5.
6. Candib LM. Medicine and the family: a feminist perspective. New York: HarperCollins Publishers, Basic Books; 1995.
7. Silver MP, Hamilton AD, Biswas A, Warrick NI. A systematic review of physician retirement planning. Hum Resour Health. 2016;14(1):67.

8. Onyura B, Leslie K. In reply to Auster. Acad Med. 2016;91(3):289–90.
9. Onyura BP, Bohnen JMD, Wasylenki DMD, et al. Reimagining the self at late-career transitions: how identity threat influences academic physicians' retirement considerations. Acad Med. 2015;90(6):794–801.
10. Kalet AL, Fletcher KE, Ferdman DJ, Bickell NA. Defining, navigating, and negotiating success: the experiences of mid-career Robert wood Johnson clinical scholar women. J Gen Intern Med. 2006;21(9):920–5.
11. Feller A. Termination. Panel report. J Am Psychoanal Assoc. 2009;57(5):1185–95.
12. Viorst J, Cruz RI. Alexander and the terrible, horrible, no good, very bad day. New York: Simon & Schuster; 1972.
13. Viorst J. Experiences of loss at the end of analysis: the analyst's response to termination. Psychoanal Inq. 1982;2(3):399–418.
14. Carmichael LP. The family in medicine, process or entity? J Fam Pract. 1976;3(5):562–3.

Chapter 9
Retiring or Just Tiring?

Barry G. Saver

Editors' Introduction

Barry Saver not only said goodbye to many clinical sites during his career, mostly not by his own choice, but also to the hundreds, if not thousands, of patients whom he cared for at those locations and to the colleagues with whom he shared his ebullient sense of humor, his wonderful stories, and his extensive and critical knowledge of prevention in primary care. I (LMC) was one of those fortunate colleagues; I had the pleasure of sharing an office with him for most of his time in Massachusetts. Barry conveys his deep sense of caring for friends and patients through his presence and his ability to listen and respond, whatever the issue. His intolerance of bureaucratic obstacles to doing the right thing in medical care and medical institutions makes him that unusual person who says what he thinks rather than what people want to hear. And he always has a story of a worst-case scenario caused by greed, arrogance, or stupidity to top whatever catastrophe you can tell him about!

I think I surprised myself when I decided to officially retire as a family doctor at the ripe old age of 66. I had always assumed that, barring something forcing me to stop, I would work until at least 70 and probably longer. "I like what I do," I thought. "Why would I want to retire?" Besides, retiring would mean no more income from work, which to someone who grew up in the depression seemed almost inconceivable. (No, I'm not old enough to have grown up in the Great Depression, but my father did and never recovered from it and my siblings and I grew up in his depression.) So it was a real struggle to even think about retiring, let alone decide to do it. How and why did I get there? As you'd expect, it was from a combination of factors, some internal and some external.

B. G. Saver (✉)
Swedish Cherry Hill Family Medicine Residency, Seattle, WA, USA

Department of Family Medicine, Emeritus, University of Washington, Seattle, WA, USA

I attended a medical school that did not even have a family medicine department or any longitudinal experience opportunities, so I knew nothing of continuity until my residency. I had no preparation for saying goodbye to patients I had gotten to know for up to 3 years when I was finishing residency. It was painful, but the limited timeframe of residency was known to my patients as well as to me from the start. The goodbye had to happen, and it did.

I left my first job, at a community health center (CHC), quite abruptly after being there less than 2 years. The second time I declined to become medical director, after the second time the clinic's current medical director quit because of our administration's dishonesty and incompetence, I also submitted my resignation, so there was little time for grieving and little opportunity to say goodbye to patients. The clinic's multilevel dysfunction also meant that there were fewer patients with whom I'd had an ongoing relationship with enough contact to develop strong bonds.

That job made me think I should go do a fellowship to get research training so I could do the research to show how stupid and evil the health care system was that was making it so hard for my CHC patients to get appropriate specialty care, even if they had Medicaid, and how harmful it was to leave so many people uninsured. (E.g., "Oh, sorry, doctor doesn't set bones on MediCal patients.") That led directly to my first two major medical career failures. First, I left graduate school in chemistry to go to medical school, become a family doctor, work with patients struggling to obtain access to health care, and never do research again. Oops. Second, it took me some years to realize my utter naïveté—there was already plenty of relevant research, and it was a political, not a research, issue. Whatever research I did was not going to make universal health insurance happen. Or even eliminate health care inequities based on race, socioeconomic status, or language spoken.

But that decision did mean that, when I took my next job, I expected I'd be leaving in a year. That job was working at the organization that developed the model for PACE (Program of All-Inclusive Care for the Elderly), and most of my patients had moderate to severe dementia and spoke Cantonese or Toisanese, so I did not develop many deep relationships during that year, and leaving was not too difficult. I did have one patient who taught me a lesson about the importance of continuity and relationships for patients. He had grown up in the US, spoke fluent English, and was in the program because of severe peripheral vascular disease with gangrene, not dementia. We spoke quite frequently, and when I left the program to get married and move to Seattle for a fellowship, he gave me a traditional dragon and phoenix painting he had made for us as a wedding gift. Having no easy access to art paper or canvas, he made it on a clay pot available through the program. I still have it on a shelf in our house. I was quite surprised, a few years later, to receive a letter from one of the nurses in the program. I had not known that he was her father. He had recently passed away, and she wrote me because, going through his effects, she found that he had retained a letter I had written in response to a letter he had sent me after I left. She expressed surprise and gratitude that I would have taken the time to write him back. I wrote her that responding to him had seemed totally normal as he was such a kind man and I had enjoyed being his doctor, but I was surprised to learn that this had meant enough to him that he would have retained my letter. It was a good lesson in the value of even a fairly short-term relationship with a patient.

After I completed my fellowship at the University of Washington (UW), I ended up committing my third major career mistake, taking a part-time, soft money-funded position at UW and a separate, part-time position at a community health center in West Seattle rather than a full-time position elsewhere that would have supported my research interests. Advice from people I respected was to go elsewhere, to a place that would value me, but my wife did not want to move to either of the locations that were offering me real jobs. I was asked and declined to take on the role of a medical director as I was starting at the health center. I was just working there part-time and wanted to focus on getting my research going. On my first morning there, the departing medical director had just finished his last night on call and handed me his pager, now mine. When I asked why, if he was leaving, he would even suggest I consider becoming medical director, he said something that stuck in my brain. "It's not so much where we are now as the mileage it took to get here."

I worked for several years with two part-time jobs, but in another bad career choice, I let my department at UW convince me to become full-time there, with my time at the CHC paid for by a subcontract. I agreed because there was a prestigious fellowship for which you had to be a full-time faculty member to apply. I had been told I would be the department's next candidate (applications were limited in a variety of ways). However, despite that promise, I was not allowed to apply for that fellowship the next time someone could apply. But becoming a full-time employee did give them the power to tell me (remember error #3?), after 7 years of continuity practice in the CHC, that they desperately needed me to move my practice to the residency clinic. Having been at the health center for over 7 years, I had developed deep relationships with many patients. I had been there long enough to learn that continuity sometimes really did matter, such as patients who had been utterly uninterested in quitting smoking who, after 3 or 4 years, would say, "You know, we've been talking about this for a long time. I think I'm ready to try." I made myself learn to start prescribing mood stabilizers when I had patients who clearly had bipolar disorder but either could not or would not see a psychiatrist but would take the medication if I prescribed it for them. I did what I could to help patients through crises like having a second son murdered. Saying goodbye was one of the most painful things I had done, but I wasn't ready to quit the university and take on a full-time clinical position at the health center, as I was still harboring delusions that my research could change policy to help millions of people like my patients. And being at the university for my clinic would let me teach more, something else I really loved doing and for which the opportunities had been quite limited in my previous job configuration.

However, all of 6 months after I started at the residency clinic, I was told the department now desperately needed me to help start providing family medicine services at a public health clinic (error #3 strikes again!) as part of a new relationship with the public health department, which had declared that providing primary care services was a core public health mission. As it happens, the clinic they wanted me to start was at a site 3 miles away from the health center where I had been practicing for 7 years.

I should have quit then, but I had found a good research collaborator, and we had managed to get ourselves "overunderfunded" by getting a number of shortish-term, policy-focused grants, none of which really paid for all the time required to do the work. I also had no immediate job offers in places we'd want to live, so I swallowed hard and set to work with negotiations and plans for the new family medicine clinic. Given my short tenure there, leaving the residency clinic was not too difficult. When I started at the new clinic, it was immediately made clear that all the nice talk about providing primary care and seeing children along with the pediatricians who had been providing care there for years was utter fiction. A family physician would get to see a child there only over a pediatrician's dead body. If then.

Six months later, the health department decided that, because of rising costs for providing jail health services, which was a statutory obligation, primary care was not, after all, a core public health mission, and they would be "reconfiguring to improve access," meaning closing all the family medicine clinics in 6 months and telling patients to find care elsewhere. When patients asked me what they were supposed to do, sometimes I said, "Well, if you have a serious medical problem and can't get care at a community health center or Harborview (the county hospital), you can always commit a minor crime; they have to provide you medical care in jail." So my goodbyes there were a bit different than in previous departures.

I foolishly did not quit at that point, despite my anger. The department then asked me to go to the new clinic at Harborview, where it had just started a 2-2-2 satellite residency site. Several of my closest colleagues, including my main research collaborator, who also felt strongly about working for social justice, were also there, which made a huge difference. As one might expect of a hospital co-run by a university and a public health department, the administration was a frustrating mess, but many of the staff were amazing, wonderful people. My patients came from all over—Seattle, King County, East Africa, Mexico and Central America, Southeast Asia, and more. Frequently, I could get them what they needed. Well, with the exception of orthopedic care. Somehow, even at the public hospital, the orthopedists were allowed to decline to see patients, which they almost always did with our referrals. And, curiously, despite having a separate psychiatric emergency room and a huge edifice, psychiatry was allowed to refuse to see uninsured patients once they were no longer in crisis, which meant that we were always getting new patients coming into our clinic with a brief note from psychiatry: "Dx: psychosis, NOS. Plan: please continue XXX [whichever neuroleptic drug they had been prescribed]." So I unexpectedly got to start prescribing medication for psychosis as well as bipolar disorder. I also got to precept residents who were mostly there for the mission of the program, which was a wonderful addition to my career activities.

In my research, I tried to transition to more patient-oriented studies with the hope that I could get more stability through longer-term grants that the NIH can award rather than the model of short-term, underfunded grants that was the norm for policy-focused work. But, in 2005, as grant funding hit a nadir, I went to my Chair and said, "I have 4 grant proposals pending now, but unless all are funded, I am going to be short next year and, in the current funding environment, the odds of all 4 being funded are extremely low." He looked at me and said, "Well, you've got a problem." So much for having spent over 14 years on faculty there, bringing in grant funding to support nearly all of my nonclinical time.

So, I looked for a new job. I severely limited my options by only considering positions that would both offer support for trying to continue to do research and let me work in a safety net setting, ideally in a location where my family would feel comfortable living. I eventually accepted a position at UMass Medical School. Leaving my academic department was not too hard; I had a few good friends and colleagues I would really miss, but people coming and going is an expected part of life, and we could stay in touch. Leaving my clinic at Harborview was more complicated. I had a love-hate relationship with it. I loved most of my patients there, whom I had gotten to know for up to 7 years. I loved many of the staff, who were there for the mission. And I hated the inescapable administrative idiocy that was compounded by the joint management by two large bureaucratic organizations. I hated the terrible Cerner EMR ("EHR" or "electronic health record" is purely a marketing term; "EBR" for "electronic billing record" would be most accurate) that UW had bought because it was allegedly top-of-the-line for inpatient computerized order entry and then rolled out first for outpatient care, where it made our work harder and our workdays longer.

This was not the first time I had to say goodbye to patients I had cared for over many years, including many with whom I had never spoken beyond a simple greeting without an interpreter, but it was harder, partly because of a spillover from my feelings about why I was leaving, but not all. I was truly touched when I noticed that the modal statement from my patients was, "Thank you for listening." This was my first real affirmation that some patients, at least, had understood what I was doing and why I was almost always running late. And they valued it enough to put up with it.

Here, I should note that I have never been a "fast" provider. I have joked that I should change my last name legally to "Saver-I'm-sorry-I'm-late" just to get that out of the way up front. But, having spent virtually all my career working in the safety net, I never felt comfortable with the "Sorry, we just have time for 1 problem, you'll have to make another appointment for that" approach to care as I never had confidence my patient could and would come back at a predictable time in the future. If they needed something important now, I wanted to do it now. So, I always ran behind and finished the clinic late. In the days of handwritten charts, it was not so bad as my history and physical were written in the room, so maybe I left the clinic at 6:00 or 6:30 when colleagues left at 5:30 or 6:00. When I had to switch to dictation, it got worse as the writing in the room was only notes for my dictation, so I had to repeat that work. Being an academic with just a part-time clinical practice gave me the flexibility to pay this tax in my free time to be able to provide care respectfully to my patients. I don't think I could have sustained it for long had I been in full-time clinical practice.

I got to UMass and found that, unlike UW, social justice and care for the underserved were core missions of the department, not just a small section. I worked on developing new research projects/collaborations, did a little medical student teaching, and started practicing and precepting residents at the Family Health Center of Worcester (FHCW), an affiliated teaching health center. About one-third of my visits were in Spanish, with no interpreter. Caribbean Spanish. I should note that, while I had been "the Spanish-speaking provider" a couple of times in my career, I took French in school and my Spanish, after an 8 week, one-evening-a-week medical Spanish elective in medical school, was all picked up on the job and from looking at an introductory Spanish text to figure out some basic verb conjugation. I acquired a good technical vocabulary and the grammar of, at best, a 2-year old. Caribbean Spanish is spoken much more rapidly than Mexican/Central American Spanish and has very different slang. "La guagua???" Oh, the bus. I had to ask patients to slow down, repeat things, and explain things. But they were incredibly gracious, thanking me for speaking Spanish at all. After a few weeks, I got used to the rapid pace of speech and, to my astonishment, discovered I could, somehow, type a note in English into the EMR while conversing in Spanish. Some of my patients even got comfortable enough to correct me when I made a mistake, for which I thanked them. I had one patient who was fluently bilingual, so he knew exactly how bad my Spanish was. Yet he told me, "When it's my health, I prefer to speak in Spanish." One day, I was even farther behind than usual, and when I rushed into the room, I started speaking to him in English. He responded. But, after a minute, he said, "I thought we were going to speak in Spanish about my health." There was another patient, a Salvadoran woman in her mid-thirties. I had done a vaginal exam and seen that a Bartholin's gland cyst had recurred despite appropriate treatment. I said I wanted to refer her to gynecology for definitive treatment. She asked me if that would affect her chances of getting pregnant. I said no, it was a totally different area and could not, but I was puzzled why she had asked. She then proceeded to tell me how, before she had fled El Salvador, one day her 13-year-old daughter had just disappeared. I asked if she had heard anything about what had happened to her. "No. Esto pasa en mi país." ("This happens in my country.") I asked if she had told anyone else here about this, and she said no. I asked why, despite my bad Spanish, she had told me. She responded that she just felt she could trust me. I don't think that would have happened with an interpreter. My patients have taught me how important it is to try—even knowing just a few words of their native language makes a huge difference.

Alas, a familiar theme repeated itself at the FHCW—I loved my patients and got exposed to yet more cultures—Puerto Rican, Dominican, Albanian, Brazilian, Ghanaian, Liberian, Bhutanese, and more. I loved most of my coworkers. And I hated the administrative dysfunction, along with the EMR the FHCW had acquired My favorite online review of this EMR was quite succinct, "Friends don't let friends buy NextGen."

Separate from my job and UMass and my love/hate relationship with my clinic, I had learned, to my surprise, when I left Denver for the northeast for college, then graduate school, then medical school, that in some way I was really a westerner. The landscape spoke to me in a way eastern landscapes, despite their lushness and the much more colorful birds, did not. I found the elitist culture at the schools I went to alienating. So I decided to apply for residency only out west and never planned to live in the East again. UMass and Worcester, thankfully, were not like Yale and New Haven, Harvard and Boston, and Columbia and New York City. But I hated the cold winters and got neuropathic injuries to my big toes every winter due to Raynaud's. I had also finally figured out how the "successful research career" game worked, something none of my alleged mentors in Seattle had ever discussed with me. I could then project that the arc of my research career was not going to change enough from any future study I did, regardless of its findings, to the point where policymakers would pay any attention to my work. My research was rarely cited, even in papers to which it was directly relevant, because I had not understood that I had to become known in some specific area before people would be likely to pay any attention to what I did. So when I saw an ad by a community-based residency in Seattle seeking a faculty member with a passion for evidence-based medicine and social justice, I thought, "Hmm – that describes me. If I stay here until I retire, I'd want to move away and we'd have to get reestablished somewhere new. We loved living in Seattle and still have friends there now. I'd be happy living there after I retire. But I'd have to throw in the towel on "big R" research; it's a community-based residency. I agonized privately for weeks, not wanting to even discuss it with my wife, as UW had jerked me around about possible jobs a couple of times since we had left, and I did not want to raise and dash her hopes again. I finally decided to send off a letter of inquiry, discussing why I was certainly not a typical applicant but why I was interested and they might be interested in me. After a few months, that letter led to an interview and a job offer. The position that had been advertised had been filled shortly before I sent my letter, but a couple of pieces had been put together to make a part-time job that they expected could become full-time in the coming year.

Leaving UMass was far harder than leaving UW. I had set up a meeting with my direct supervisor, Linda, to tell her of my decision to leave, but she had gotten held up in traffic, and I ended up having to tell her my decision and explain it over the phone. Fifteen minutes later, the Chair walked into my office and sat down. "I just spoke with Linda," he said. He went on to say that, based on what she had told him, he didn't think there was anything he could do to get me to stay but, if there was, he wanted me to tell him what it was. If I never wanted to write another research grant proposal, that was fine; there were lots of things he'd love for me to do there. The contrast with "Well, you've got a problem" could not have been starker. I would be leaving a group of colleagues who shared my mission and for whom I had deep respect and affection.

Saying goodbye to patients in the clinic was, if anything, harder, too. I had been there for 9 years, longer than I had been anywhere else in my career. I had been pained by the feeling that relationships with my monolingual Spanish-speaking patients were less deep/rich than with patients with whom I spoke English because casual chit-chat in Spanish was very effortful for me, but it didn't seem to affect how they felt about me when we discussed my upcoming departure. And, again, the modal comment from patients was an expression of appreciation that I listened to them.

In addition to an even greater understanding of the value of continuity, my time in Worcester also gave me a growing understanding that sometimes we can have a deep impact in a single visit. I saw a young woman patient of a colleague whom I deeply respected. The woman had been struggling with a significant mental health issue for years. A few weeks later, my colleague asked me, "What did you say to her?" I said that I didn't remember exactly but had just tried to help her move forward. I queried why she had asked. She told me that the patient told her that I had helped her more in that one visit than 10 years of seeing therapists. I sure wish I remembered what I had said! There was another patient, a man in his 30s or 40s, with an appointment for a URI. But when I came into the room and put out my hand to shake his, he held back. I inquired about that, and, as I suspected, he had severe OCD. I asked if he was in therapy, and he said he had been for years. I asked for details of the therapy and it was clear it was not exposure-response prevention (ERP) therapy, the flavor of CBT (cognitive behavioral therapy) with demonstrated efficacy for OCD. I suggested he might want to change therapists to one who knew ERP and described some basic exercises to start with. He grew teary and said, "You mean this can really get better?" About a month later, a nurse knocked on the door of the exam room I was in to say that there was a patient on the phone who wanted to talk with me right then and said it was important. So, I left the room and picked up the phone. It was that man, who wanted me to know that he was out hiking in the forest, getting his hands dirty, and was fine with that. A month or so later, he was on my schedule, having made me his PCP. When I walked in, I hesitated to reach out to shake his hand, not wanting to make him uncomfortable. He shoved his hand at me and said, "It's fine, doc. I can shake your hand." And then, a week or two before I left the clinic, I was walking down the hall between rooms when a young woman stopped me. She said, "Dr. Saver? You probably don't remember me, but I just wanted to thank you for what you did last year when you saw me. God has put you here to do this and you have to keep helping people." My first thought was that this was a put-up job by colleagues trying to get me to change my mind. But I looked around and there was nobody in sight. I finally remembered that I had seen her for something. I couldn't remember what, but she had mentioned being really scared by the planned surgery scheduled for a couple of months later in Boston. I think it was eye surgery, maybe for keratoconus, and she was afraid she'd end up blind. I had just tried to reassure her.

Those anecdotes are not meant to suggest I think I am anything special. I think we all have times where we can make a critical difference for a patient, as long as we are willing to listen and be present. I am going to miss that opportunity when I retire, too.

I never told my colleagues at my new job in Seattle that it WAS my retirement job—no more chasing grant funding, just teach and see patients, two things I loved doing. When I got to Swedish, the program director told me that, well, actually, it might not be possible to get me up to full time in the coming year. After the initial shock, I decided I was fine working 70% of the time. However, continuing in the theme of failure, it turned out I couldn't even fail out of research successfully. After I had accepted the job but while I was still at UMass, the NIH put out a request for applications that was the closest thing I had seen to a possible funding mechanism for an idea I had been trying to get funded for several years, so I wrote a proposal and got an R01 grant funded after I arrived in Seattle. So, 70% became 90%.

I had thought hard about taking this job in part because it was at a private, non-profit hospital and within a Catholic-based hospital system, though technically part of a secular hospital system. But the hospital had formerly been a Catholic charity hospital that provided care to patients from all the CHCs, insured or not, and had been founded to provide care to Seattle's African American community and to other patients shunned by the other hospitals. I had admitted patients there when I was working at the CHC in West Seattle, and, unlike the community hospital near my first CHC job, they never once asked me, "What is the patient's insurance?" when I called about an admission. The residency program had a long history of training clinicians to work with the underserved, and a majority of the residents were now based in CHCs for their continuity clinics. Due to the Hyde Amendment, none of my CHC jobs had allowed providing pregnancy termination services, and the residents did get that training elsewhere. So, I figured I could deal with the ownership issues.

My colleagues here, too, were amazing people. In my time here, the program made a very intentional decision to focus on recruiting residents who come from the populations we serve—BIPOC and LGBTQI+. At this point, I am an outlier as a white/cis/straight male. My patients include African Americans who, even if they have been forced by gentrification to live far away, still come to this hospital because it was there for them, their parents, and maybe their grandparents. Because we are located near Seattle's gayborhood, I have a large number of gay male patients, particularly older men, who I think feel more comfortable with a male clinician, and I am one of the very few such in the clinic these days. I have East African patients, like I did at Harborview. And a few West African patients, reminding me that while my grammar in French is much better than in Spanish, my medical vocabulary is all Spanish. I am truly grateful for all the opportunities my career has given me to get to know such a diversity of people, appreciate our common humanity, and overcome prejudices acquired in childhood.

I had not anticipated encountering any of my old patients at Swedish, but that has happened, too. Harborview is only a few miles away, so they draw patients from the same area. One time, I walked into a room with a resident to examine a Somali patient he had presented. The patient looked at me and exclaimed, "I know you! You were my first doctor, at Harborview, when I first came to this country! I was going to leave this clinic, but now I will stay." Another time I went in with a resident, having recognized the name of an old patient who had severe, hard-to-control hypertension and an opiate use disorder. When she was my patient at Harborview, she had been doing well, working, raising her daughter, and being stable on methadone maintenance. But then she lost her insurance, couldn't afford methadone treatment, and relapsed onto street opiates. She had told me how she had gotten hooked, "I was 18 and a friend just said to try this. I did it once and it opened a door I could never close." Here she was, over 10 years later, still struggling with opiates and blood pressure. She looked at me, recognized me, and turned to the resident. "You know what I like about him? He listens."

So, how could I possibly decide to retire? Many things contributed. I have gotten reminders that none of us lives forever, with my brother passing away the summer before last. COVID canceled his bucket list trip to the Galapagos and Machu Picchu on which I was going to accompany him. Now that will never happen. Friends are starting to get diagnosed with fatal conditions. On the other hand, COVID will seriously limit ideas of "retire and travel." But the bigger piece comes from my work environment. Our hospital administration apparently decided that they had had enough of training residents to work in the safety net and wanted us and our "sister residency" (located less than a mile away) to focus on producing graduates who would work for them in their clinics. How that was supposed to work when over half of our residents had their clinics in CHCs was a mystery to me. Both program directors resigned and the administration conducted a prolonged, expensive search, at the end of which they rejected the two remaining strong and viable candidates," both faculty from the programs who believed in their social justice-focused missions. I was planning to quit the week we had a last-second meeting with the system CEO, who declared that he supported the mission of the programs and did not care if our graduates went to work for the system; what mattered was whether we were serving the needs of our community. I held off on my resignation letter, and his words were followed by actions, so I did not quit. However, this process led to the loss of two valued colleagues, along with the earlier loss of our program director.

A second part of the "remake the residency program" was putting our clinic under the purview of their medical group that runs their community-based clinics. They had no understanding of how our jobs as residency faculty differed from the clinicians they employed in their clinics and insisted that rather than being salaried for essentially all our work and making our schedules fit the program's needs, our precepting and personal clinic time would be set by contract and payment would be productivity-based. Oh, and we also needed to sign the contracts, which we hadn't had for 2 years, immediately. We rejected that and they rejected our counteroffer, so all the faculty in both residencies hired legal representation and, after spending over $5000 each, we finally agreed to a contract pretty much the same as our initial counteroffer, allowing for people to stay on salary for up to a couple of years before they had to switch to productivity payment. "The mileage to get there" is certainly playing a role in my decision now.

I changed over to productivity-based compensation a few months back and I think I am being paid a few thousand dollars more a year. Does that make me happier? Not in the slightest. I have no control over my scheduling, or who shows up, so if I am coding appropriately for what I do, I actually have no control over my "productivity." If I, or my colleagues, were motivated by potential for higher income, I don't think we'd be in family medicine or residency teaching, nor would most of us have worked in CHCs. I would happily be less "productive" and, if necessary, get paid less, if I could control my clinic scheduling and limit it to what I thought would let me attend appropriately to my patients' needs. Instead, I find myself dreading clinic as I review my upcoming schedule and figure out what things I hope to get addressed. Once I am actually in clinic, seeing patients, I am happy (except for feeling time pressure), but the dysphoric anticipation has been wearing on me.

I also need to mention the steadily increasing pressure to achieve "quality metrics," e.g., proportions of patients up to date on immunizations, mammograms, breast cancer screening, colon cancer screening, and depression screening. This is not unique to my setting; these are standard measures because there are simple guidelines recommending them and they are easily captured as binary data from the EMR. I find this quite demoralizing. It's not that I don't believe in the value of most of these measures, but virtually none of them needs **me** to get them done; they could be accomplished by a proactive system. The only time I ought to be involved is when a patient is refusing an important service and I can help them reconsider their refusal. Should my quality as a clinician be judged by such measures? Should my pay depend on them when they are fundamentally system issues? And do not get me started on Press-Ganey satisfaction surveys and the like. Google tells me their response rate is about 16.5%, meaning they have no statistical validity at all. I could never get a paper published with a response rate like that. Being judged by meaningless and/or invalid measures is remarkably dispiriting.

Finally, I should mention the role the EMR has played. At Swedish, we use Epic, one of the least disliked EMRs. (The EMR user satisfaction scale seems to run from "loathe" to "dislike.") When COVID hit, in-person visits nearly disappeared and video and phone visits became possible, which in many cases was appropriate and much more convenient for patients. Communication through the EMR also jumped substantially. Most care has now returned to in-person visits, but EMR volume has not dropped back. For many patient inquiries, I could respond, "Please set up an appointment," but if it is relatively straightforward, I usually try to take care of it. That's how I would hope to be treated as a patient. Why shouldn't I treat my patients the same way? We are told that such portal-based interactions may become (modestly) billable, and, honestly, I don't really want that. I don't want to be like a lawyer where every interaction is billable; it creates barriers to patients seeking care when they think they need it. I view piecemeal fee-for-documentation payment as a root cause of much of our health care system's dysfunction. I really have no interest in wasting cognitive effort on learning and applying the latest CPT-4 coding guidelines (Current Procedural Terminology, Fourth Edition) and teaching that to residents; I do it now because I have to. If I were practicing in a setting where I was responsible for the care of a reasonably sized panel of patients, and we interacted by whatever means seemed most appropriate, from office visit to portal message, and I didn't have to waste time thinking about billing, would I be retiring now? Probably not. The closest thing to that, direct primary care, has no appeal to me since it's not an option for most of the patients I went into medicine to serve.

One thing caught me by surprise this time, as I say goodbye to patients, that makes it substantially less painful than I had anticipated—the amazing grace and gratitude they have displayed. Yes, there are tears and pleas to stay on. But I did not anticipate that so many patients, including those for whom retirement before disability or death is just a pipe dream, being so gracious. Again and again, I am congratulated, told I had earned a good retirement, asked if I had any plans for what I will do, and been wished well. This really caught me by surprise. While it has made saying goodbye somewhat less difficult, it has made me realize more how much I will be missing soon.

Chapter 10
Shy But Not Retiring

Kurt C. Stange

Editors' Introduction

The sun rarely rises before Kurt Stange. Its first rays of light will find him silently meditating in a chair near a window. Don't be fooled by the title of his essay. He is shy but not so shy to avoid greeting a stranger on the bus or along the bike path or at a meeting. At any given moment, he may have more active mentees than anyone else we know. Kurt's generosity and curiosity exceed his shyness. He retires early every evening unless a friend requests his company. And when not sleeping or meditating, his body moves—pacing, walking, biking, or on the treadmill by his computer. Kurt's life represents a study in living within the tension between action and reflection. It wasn't always this way.

Kurt Stange began his vocation steadily, accumulating the signs of academic success and an illustrious career through getting NIH (National Institute of Health) grants, multiple publications, keynote address invitations, promotions, and awards. He became the founding editor of the Annals of Family Medicine. But, deep down, niggles of doubt appeared, and his close friends could feel it. Change was already happening. Always passionate about relationships, the importance of place, and seeking understanding of the magic underlying family medicine, he struggled for more peace of mind. He learned that means matter more than outcomes. Then came the sabbatical and real transformation started happening. The essay that follows tells this story. The importance of relationships surfaces repeatedly, especially the relationship with self. Letting go may be the most difficult part of saying goodbye.

I'm shy. But I'm not retiring. Once, however, I did take a year-long foray into retirement. During that sabbatical year and in its impact on the 15 years since, a few lessons, potentially pertinent to retirement and relationships, have surfaced.

K. C. Stange (✉)
Center for Community Health Integration, Case Western Reserve University, Cleveland, OH, USA
e-mail: kcs@case.edu

© The Author(s), under exclusive license to Springer Nature Switzerland AG 2023
L. M. Candib, W. L. Miller (eds.), *Family Doctors Say Goodbye*, https://doi.org/10.1007/978-3-031-33654-6_10

I learned that stepping away from an occupation, like many life transitions, is sometimes chosen and sometimes forced upon us. My temporary retirement was a bit of both.

I learned about:

balancing action with reflection,
    investing in old and new relationships,
    taking time to create space for new learning and meaning,
    detaching from the outcomes of actions,
    being open to emergence in the face of uncertainty, and
    preparing to let go.

Balancing Action with Reflection

Like most Americans, I'm pretty action-oriented. Since finishing my residencies in family medicine, preventive medicine, and public health, I'd spent 19 years in a continuity family practice. After 5 years, I stopped delivering babies to make more time for research and teaching but kept on seeing patients in the office, hospital, emergency department, nursing home, and home as a member of the practice of the residency program at University Hospitals of Cleveland, where I'm on the faculty at Case Western Reserve University.

The biggest professional joys and much-needed support for the low points involved developing teams of colleagues who felt like fellow outcasts from the mainstream of academic and big system medicine but kindred spirits with the hearts of the generalist healer. Together, we tried to balance garnering enough conventional success to put bread on the table and to create space for the unconventional work that might make a difference while not selling out to the seductive trappings of mainstream success in an increasingly dysfunctional health care system.

After some rough patches, our research managed to find ways to wedge the expansiveness of family medicine into the narrowness of categorical funding mechanisms. While whirling through that often-uncomfortable dance, my colleagues and I developed multiple practice-based research networks, transdisciplinary collaborations, and observational and intervention studies to try to understand and improve generalist practice. After multiple initial failures, we managed to get external funding for our work, which gave us some autonomy to study the care of whole people while being funded to study their diseases. We never cracked the *New England Journal of Medicine*, but were able to publish, in family medicine and related journals, work that felt like it started to recognize what is important about family medicine [1]. Teams of colleagues became friends, and we helped each other grow personally as well as professionally. To create a mainstream platform for our outsider work, I became the cancer center's founding associate director for population and prevention research, and director of a multisite family practice and primary care research center, both of which supported vital infrastructure and relationships.

The patient care, teaching, and research felt meaningful and, over time, adapted both to a crazy culture that rewards overextension and to my enabling inner striving for credibility. I called on my skill learned in residency—of getting by on not enough sleep—often going back to the office after the children were in bed and ignoring my tendency to become impatient when sleep deprived.

My wife, Anne, and I juggled family and careers. She had multiple career transitions—each stressful in the moment but, in retrospect, each was handled with grace. After some childcare arrangements that worked only in the short term, we were blessed to find someone who became part of our family. Our two children were developing well, despite a couple of public instances when we wished their physician parents hadn't taught them the correct anatomic names for body parts.

But the plate felt too full. Or rather, I felt like there were a dozen disparate dishes, and I was a circus performer, running between them, twirling each plate on its own stick, frantically scurrying to keep them all spinning so the whole complex didn't crash to the ground. It seemed like all the plates together somehow created their own sustaining gravitational field so that if I let one drop, the entire enterprise would collapse. I felt trapped as much by my successes as by my failures.

In this crazy space, an absurd idea emerged:
Faculty members can take sabbaticals.
I'm a faculty member!

The university handbook says that after 7 years, faculty members can apply for 6 months away with full pay or a whole year at half pay. At that point, I had 17 years under my belt.

But what about my patients? I can't leave my patients. What about my family? They can't leave their busy lives while I take a year off. What about the momentum I had struggled to build? Would I be able to get that back if I took a year away?

I stayed in that state of uncertainty and ongoing overextension for another year. Then the "can'ts" started fading, and I began dreaming about a year-long sabbatical that would allow multiple roles and projects to end but would keep enough going to pay for the half of my salary not covered by the university. I would give up my cancer center leadership role. I would take a year away from my dependency on my patients and my sense that they were dependent on me. Perhaps I could start when our younger child goes away to college. Since my wife couldn't leave her job, maybe I could spend half my time in town and take two forays out of the country for 2–3 months each and have her join me in the middle of each for a vacation.

But faculty members in the college of arts and sciences take sabbaticals. Medical school faculty members don't. The only other medical school faculty member I'd ever heard of taking a sabbatical never returned. And was I really going to give up my practice for a year?

I secretly selected a start date shortly after our daughter's high school graduation but was still uncertain and uncommitted. I told only a few people about my sabbatical dream. I kept spinning all the plates.

Then I got an email from a mentor, Larry Green, in Denver. It said,

Yesterday, Margie and I were driving across West Texas, which gives one a chance to loosen (?lose) one's mind. I started thinking about all the things you are involved in nationally, and on your local scene. Do you see a way to make it safely to your sabbatical? Anything your friends can do to help?

Three days later, I got a box in the mail from my father. In his retirement in Arizona, he'd started making beautiful wooden bowls. The box contained a flat bowl with a wood-burned image in the center. The image was of a candle, oriented sideways, with a wick and a flame coming out of each end. Wood-burned around the edge of the bowl were the letters D. B. T. C. A. B. E. I didn't have to spell it out to know that the letters stood for *Don't burn the candle at both ends.*

I hadn't been communicating frequently with either my father or Larry. And I certainly hadn't been telling them about my sense of overextension. The fact that in the same week they'd both intuited my urgent need for a change gave me the resolve to take my sabbatical. I put in the formal application to the university and, still striving for legitimacy, started working on two stories—one story for myself about rejuvenation, another for my work masters about enhancing my productivity on the treadmill when I returned.

Sabbatical and sabbath have the same word root. After decades of working 7 days a week, I decided that my sabbatical would involve taking 1 day a week for reflection and rejuvenation. I decided to start a journal, making a short entry each evening, and a longer reflection each sabbath day.

The sabbatical was approved but without any financial support. So, I kept a few grant-funded projects going, planning to do some intensive work during bursts at the beginning, middle, and end but promoting others to handle the day-to-day work while I was away. I'd written the sabbatical into an application for a professorship from the American Cancer Society, and in a miracle of timing and good fortune, it was funded to start on my first day of sabbatical, supporting most of the other half of my salary.

The first sabbatical day was a Sunday. After a dawn bike ride with my daughter, mowing the lawn, and lunch with my family, I opened a new Word file, named it *Sabbatical Journal*, and typed July 1, 2007. Then I wondered, "How do you write a journal?"

What poured out in the ensuing hours of tearful typing were pages of gratitude. Gratefulness for the many ways that the house of cards my life had become had tottered but not crumbled. Thankfulness for the many ways I'd been rescued from such a collapse—Carlos Jaén stepping up to lead the National Demonstration Project for the Patient-Centered Medical Home, for which, working from the end of my rope, I had become ineffectual. Before that, my mentor and colleague Eva Kahana stepping up to combine and lead two large research projects that were coming due for renewal at the same time. Before that, Larry Green stepping up to take on the Prescription for Health Initiative I was supposed to lead for the Robert Wood Johnson Foundation, so that instead (with several other colleagues joining in), I could take on the new role of editor of the *Annals of Family Medicine*.

While reflecting every day in my sabbatical journal, I started asking what is important. What are my opportunities to make a positive difference in the world?

What personal practices do I need to be effective at that? I started reading more broadly and meeting with more diverse people than I'd grown accustomed to. I used Sundays to be present in nature and to think bigger thoughts, but mostly to try to open myself, to get over myself, and to listen to what the Universe was trying to tell me.

Investing in Old and New Relationships

There is never a convenient time for a sabbatical. (I don't know if the same is true for an actual retirement but look forward to reading the rest of the stories in this book to find out.)

But taking a year off and being away just as both children went away to college seemed like a well-timed move. What didn't seem like a good move was to say to my wife, "Hey, honey, great raising the kids with you. Now I'm outa here for a year. See ya!"

I included Anne in the sabbatical planning, of course. The planned summer at home with the whole family was bonding, perhaps because we all sensed that we'd never be together again in quite the same way. After dropping the young adults off at college, Anne and I immediately flew to the Yorkshire Dales for a two-week hiking vacation. Then I dropped her off at Heathrow to fly home and took the train to Cambridge, where I would spend the Michaelmas Term as an Overseas Visiting Scholar at St. John's College. After that, we had a family reunion at home for Christmas, and then Anne and I had January as empty nesters before I headed off to New Zealand. Anne had banked her vacation, and we had a magical 3-week holiday on the South and the North Islands in the middle of my time there. And then I spent a quiet final 3 months of sabbatical back home in Cleveland.

The most important thing I did, and I did this based on a strong voice from inside rather than from any planning, was to, in my heart, re-commit to the marriage. With the children leaving, it would have been a transition even without the sabbatical. But changing work at the same time as changing our major family focus forced me to think about which relationships were important. The marriage to Anne was top of the list, and that subtle, silent recommitment manifested in thousands of little thoughts that became hundreds of words and dozens of actions that, over time, developed a powerful message that, fortunately for me, was reciprocated.

My journal reflects gratitude for the compounding interest of investing in banks of relationships, with the marriage being the foundation.

Other connections were more complex to (re)invest in. For many of my colleagues, my going away for a year felt more like abandonment—a withdrawal from the relationship bank rather than a deposit.

I'd already experienced blowback from some of my patients 14 years earlier, when I'd stopped delivering babies. From one newly pregnant mother of two, "What do you mean you *stopped*? Start up again!" Sharing critical life events with patients is one of the privileges of being a physician. For a family physician, that intimacy creates a sense of obligation to invest the interest from the resulting relationship bank back into a healing connection by being there for future events and family members.

Before starting the sabbatical, I'd gotten a list of all the patients I'd seen at least once in the past 5 years and sorted it by the number of encounters. But since we physicians are notoriously bad at knowing which of our encounters with which patients make a difference in their lives, I'd sent a letter to almost everyone letting them know of my plans for being away for a year and inviting them to take advantage of extra patient care slots added to my schedule to accommodate conversations about transitions.

As I anticipate reading in other chapters in this book, patients as a group can be incredibly gracious when physicians cry out for self-care for themselves after they've seen us put our needs in the background to tend to theirs. It was validating and rewarding for me, and often, I hope, helpful for patients/families, to recollect important shared moments, answer questions or make changes one or both of us had been putting off, or consider a substitute physician for the year. One patient, a postal worker with whom I'd shared many personal and family health events and whom I'd talked down from buying a gun and "going postal" during a particularly dehumanizing episode at work, brought me a blank leather-bound journal and a pen—even though I hadn't mentioned my plan to journal. Several patients who'd moved on to other physicians for insurance or other reasons reconnected, often, I believe, for the chance to be witnessed again by another human being who had shared a crisis or a joy. A few patients were angry; many were wistful; and some, of course, didn't make contact.

I was gratified to reciprocate those who came in to feel the personal connection as well as to meet instrumental needs. I confess to having felt relieved to hand off some of those who came in with long lists of hard-to-meet requests. For the few that were angry and for those who didn't show up, I tried hard to discern, sop up, and reconcile the roots of prior abandonments, to dig into my own healthy and unhealthy attachments, and to plant some seeds for future growth for us both. I tried to soften things by planning to return, not knowing then, or even allowing myself to consider that I might end up going in a different direction.

In another kind of intimate relationship, my colleagues in the Center for Research in Family Medicine & Primary Care had already been upset at my diminishing ability to hold things together and to get work done between meetings. When I announced my sabbatical, their anger reached a boil, using the F-bomb as an adjective before the word sabbatical. Before announcing it to the group, however, I'd had a quiet conversation with one of the leaders, Carlos Jaén. Carlos too had been overly busy, having taken on a department chair role that reduced his ability to be directly involved in some of our center's research work. As I'd later note with gratitude during the first day of sabbatical journaling, he quietly agreed to step up to lead the National Demonstration Project for the Patient-Centered Medical Home. The others were skeptical, but he ended up doing a phenomenal job, far better than I would have done, and I enjoyed the ability to step far into the background under his leadership. When we see each other now, after we catch up on our children's lives, he thanks me for rejuvenating his research career with this opportunity. I thank him for saving my life by keeping me from falling into the abyss.

When I met with my Center colleagues near the sabbatical midpoint (between my time away in England and New Zealand) and told them about all the parts of my day job I was still doing remotely, they became incensed on my behalf. Having invested their time to free me up for a sabbatical, they insisted that I do more to really get away. As a result, several of them and the other editors stepped up to let me take 3 months away from my role as editor of the *Annals of Family Medicine*. Without that break, I probably would have resigned within a year or two. But the time away and the team solidarity rejuvenated my sense of purpose in that work, and I ended up continuing service as an editor for another decade.

Taking Time to Create Space for New Learning and Meaning

Everyone had told me that I needed to leave town right away for my sabbatical, or nothing would change. But as word got out about my planned time away, the phone started ringing a bit less, as people apparently assumed I wouldn't want to be bothered with new opportunities or day-to-day drama. (They were right.)

During the summer home with my family, each of them had day jobs, so I started going into the office most days to tie up activities I was ending, to throw out papers and stuff that now felt more like a burden than a help, and to create space for doing something new when I returned. Wearing shorts, I biked in every day after the rush hour ended and biked home before it started up again. I had a T-shirt made that had a spiral and the word "FOCUSED" in big letters on the front. Since my desk faced away from my office door, I had a special message on the back: ON SABBATICAL. My door was always open, but the conversations framed by the T-shirt tended to be less instrumental and more about life direction and possibilities.

My sponsor at Cambridge University's St. John's College, Professor Ann Louise Kinmonth, not only provided intellectual stimulation and friendship, but the day after I arrived, she also taught me to punt—using a long pole to navigate a narrow boat up and down the River Cam. This was a treacherous endeavor on Sunday afternoons, when the river was filled with tourists. But I took to taking a punt out shortly after dawn on Sunday mornings, when the solitude of the misty river was healing. I usually followed that with in-depth, reflective journaling, church in town, then a walk along the river to the nearby town of Grantchester for lunch and some reading at the Green Man Pub, ending with the evensong service in the St. John's Chapel.

Dinner at St. John's College was like being in a Harry Potter movie. Under high ancient beams in the Great Hall, the students stood as the faculty entered in academic gowns to sit at the high table after grace was read in Latin. But my favorite meal was lunch in the 400-year-old Combination Room. The custom was to sit at the next open seat at the long oak table—kind of an academic mixer. I got good at giving a soundbite of my story and whatever critical question I was struggling with and listening to the same from the diverse people I was meeting on my right and left and across the table. The interdisciplinary intellectual ferment was incredible, and nearly every lunch produced a new book to read or a name or idea to look up as I used my sabbatical time to broaden my understanding of the generalist approach across many fields.

The rarified atmosphere of the university made me want to hang out with some regular folks. Ironically, the opportunity came from a colleague at the Cambridge University Public Health School. Bayesian biostatistician David Spiegelhalter, who has since been knighted, told me about his guilty pleasure of playing in a community samba band. I joined him, learning to play the largest drum in the band, the low surdo. We rehearsed every Wednesday night at the old Cambridge Bath House and socialized after at the White Swan Pub. During our many gigs, we put on face paint and "fancy dress" of hats, feather boas, and other visual accompaniments to music that left hundreds cheering and dancing at various fairs, the Cambridge Christmas Parade, and the Winter Frost Festival at the Tate Museum of Modern Art in London, where six dancing Elvises in white tuxedos emerged from the audience to boogie with us on stage.

On my first night in St. John's, I'd been captivated by a very different kind of music as I walked by the chapel and heard an ethereal choral sound. I became a regular at evensong and took great pleasure in the magnificent St. John's Choir, even doing a reading during the BBC broadcast of their advent services. I also became a regular at a Methodist church on the other side of town, which provided a different set of spiritual and social connections. I even dabbled in the shared solitude of a few Quaker services after a graduate student at a social event told me I must meet his advisor—a civil engineer and proud Quaker who deeply understood generalism and who set me out on very helpful interdisciplinary readings.

During the overextended years preceding the sabbatical, I had tacked an evening meditation onto my usual 30-min morning meditation routine and looked forward to having this second meditation feel like part of a slowed down sabbatical routine rather than squeezed in at the end of a hectic day. Surprisingly, the evening meditation faded away early in my mini-retirement routine. I wondered why, and then realized that I'd been using the evening meditation not for spiritual development, not to get closer to the unity of life, but to calm down at the end of days that were overpacked, revved up, and always trying to wring too much out of each minute.

In the years immediately after sabbatical, I was slow to put things back onto the schedule. For several years, I purposefully allowed myself to remain unsettled, under-scheduled, and open to what might happen next. In that liminal space, a couple of years after sabbatical, I found myself again with an evening as well as a morning meditation practice. But this time it was motivated by a deep desire from within, not by the need for a tool to enable an overextended lifestyle.

In the leisurely pace of sabbatical, I found myself more open to little acts that might make a difference in someone's life—showing patience with a new grocery checkout person and watching that goodwill spill over to the others waiting in line;

taking a personal interest in the postal clerk; sometimes reaching out to others from whom I'd become disconnected.

During the weeks before sabbatical, I had visited Miss Kunzog, my high school biology teacher and the yearbook advisor, who'd subtly opened the paths to my two careers—first in photography, then in medicine. Miss Kunzog had mentioned that the wife of the high school athletic director, who'd taught my sixth-grade religious education class, was dying of breast cancer. Later, while in Cambridge, I woke up one morning wondering what had happened and found her obituary online. Normally, I would have paused for a moment and then gone on with my day. But in the slowed-down pace of sabbatical, I decided to write an email to one of her sons, who'd been in my graduating class, and to his father, the high school athletic director. I hadn't been particularly close to either, but even if my notes didn't hit home, it was helpful to me to reflect with gratitude on the effects of their wife/mother's sixth-grade religious education teaching on my life.

After a while, I heard back from both. My classmate, now a rear admiral in the navy after his Annapolis education, reflected on how he'd heard from many people about their interactions with his mother, and it helped him to see her in a new way. I was surprised to get a hand-written letter back from the athletic director, thanking me for my kind words about his wife but also looking back with regret on all the people he'd hurt with his tough guy approach to athletics. I was awed by how my small reflections on the effects of someone fleetingly part of my life apparently caused deeper reflections on the part of people very close to her.

A few weeks later, I had another chance to use the impetus of mortality as an opportunity to reflect on the meaning in life. A former medical school and resident trainee emailed me to let me know that his father, the retired associate dean for geriatrics, who had been a mentor for me, had had a recurrence of his cancer and probably only had a few days to live. Since I was on sabbatical schedule, I delayed my trip into the office and took time to handwrite a letter and walk to the Cambridge post office, figuring that it might either arrive on time or, if not, perhaps provide some comfort to his family. And in any case, it did me good to reflect with appreciation for the effects of Dr. Amasa Ford on the field of geriatrics, on the birth of family medicine at my university, and on my career.

Ten days later, someone emailed me the front page of the local section of the Cleveland Plain Dealer, which had a long article on Dr. Ford and his passing. The article contained multiple quotations from "his colleague, Dr. Stange," regarding the effects of Dr. Ford on the field of geriatrics, on the birth of family medicine at Case Western Reserve University, and on his personal influence as a mentor. A few days later, I received an email from his son, saying the letter arrived "just in time," and he had read it out loud as his father was going in and out of consciousness. He said his father smiled, and a tear ran down his cheek. When a reporter wanted information and a source for quotations, he hoped I didn't mind that they'd given him the letter.

It gave me pause to think that on a typical pre-sabbatical day, I most likely would not have taken the time to have written these letters. And yet, on most days, whatever I would have been doing instead likely would not have been as impactful.

Experiences like this, of the openness created by slowing down and the meaning of small caring actions, helped me consider how I wanted to live when my dalliance with retirement was over.

Detaching from the Outcomes of Actions

In planning and beginning my mini-retirement, it was easy to emotionally detach from things I *wanted* to end—a cancer center leadership position; various projects for which the work now was greater than the gain; "stealth" research for which I was tired of sneaking an inclusive generalist question into reductionist funding niches; being a cog in the hamster wheel of an increasingly corporatized, top-down medical practice environment…

Negotiating the exit wasn't always easy. I'd tried to resign the cancer center leadership role 2 years earlier, but the cancer center director convinced me to stay through our renewal application to the National Cancer Center and our site visit. Those were completed just before the sabbatical, and I went to my final senior leadership meeting to let the other leaders know that, in the context of a successful 5-year renewal of the center, I was turning my position over to a highly skilled but more junior colleague, Li Li. However, having known only me in that role, the senior leaders didn't want to let go and insisted that my colleague be named *acting* associate director so that I could resume the position when I returned. I made my strongest argument about his skills being a better fit for the next phase and about not hamstringing him with the *acting* title. But they insisted on wanting me to return. The cancer center director gave me no help. Finally, I stood up and said, "I'm like Moses. I can see the promised land but can't take you there. Li is like Joshua…" and assuming a majestic pose and fixing my gaze and my outstretched arm toward the horizon, I shouted, "Li will take you – to – the – promised – land!" They looked at me like I'd gone mad. In the ensuing silence, I thanked them, gathered up my things, and quickly left the room, never to return. Sometimes it's important to manage other people's difficulties as well as your own with letting go.

Seven months into the sabbatical, I noticed a tipping point in my sense of disentanglement from the dear things and intertwined relationships that had me so overextended. I discovered that I'd become emotionally detached from everything. *I can give up everything*. Even if I'm not yet ready to give up everyone.

For me, this was the pivotal moment in the sabbatical. The sense of freedom was liberating, energizing, and a little bit scary [2].

I talked with Anne, asking permission to work part-time when I returned if I wasn't able to fully fund myself with work that was personally meaningful and that I thought had a chance to make a difference. She said yes. In the 15 years since that conversation, I haven't had to do that. But having that permission allowed me to take the risks necessary to focus on what is important rather than what is popular, what pleases others, or what gratifies my ego.

Recent years have seen some backsliding into taking on too much. But in that moment of realization during sabbatical—*I can give up everything*—and with that permission from Anne—permission that I wasn't quite ready to give myself—I started imagining a post-sabbatical life that included part-time practice and part-time unfunded writing. For the writing, I wanted to move from the dreary expository approach that I'd gotten good at using to communicate research findings toward a different way of reaching people through the heart as well as the head. Taking a writing course and attending multiple workshops, and trying my hand at narrative non-fiction, I started to find ways of telling true personal stories that seemed to complement the more cookbook approach used to tell research stories.

Despite being ready to give up everything, toward the end of the sabbatical, I realized that I didn't need to leave everything behind. Many things I'd been working on still had value; they just needed to be approached differently. In that space, I started judiciously adding back some parts of my pre-sabbatical life. But not being attached to the outcomes has clarified a goal of striving toward a more generative investment in relationships and in working on important problems that are unlikely to be resolved in my lifetime—structural racism, classism, and the devaluation and misunderstanding of generalism and the collective.

Getting some separation from ego investment in the results of my thoughts, words, and actions has also reframed my spiritual practice as more than a support for work and relationships and succeeding in the world. Rather, my spiritual practice now has primacy, and I see daily activities as fodder for spiritual development. Working toward greater discrimination and detachment from the outcomes of my actions is an important part of my effort in that spiritual practice. Detachment and the resulting peace, painfully slow movement toward selflessness, and the ability to persist in the face of defeat are also gifts of that practice. But every little bit of vacillating progress and painful backsliding makes me realize how far I am from the goal.

The ability to work on seemingly intractable problems that bruise and batter the ego may be at the root of my admiration for generalist healers who can stay in the ring with people in the messiness of life. Working toward *both* detachment from the outcome *and* connection to the sometimes-exasperating person speaks to the heart of the generalist approach that is the underpinning of being a family physician. This way of being, thinking, and doing advances the integration of the many fragmented parts of our lives toward their connection with a more encompassing whole [3].

Being Open to Emergence in the Face of Uncertainty

In the changed approach to life engendered by the sabbatical, things happened that, in retrospect, make sense. Some even look like success. But in each moment as it was lived, they felt uncertain and often looked like failure.

In the 14 years since the sabbatical, I opened myself to a new direction in community health that became clear only in fits and starts; somewhat reluctantly took on leadership roles to support a team to develop that new direction; began handing off that leadership and some of the on-the-ground work to the next generation; recommitted to my core work in generalism but approached it in a different way.

I started imagining a new direction—working more at the health care-community health interface. I looked seriously at a new job in a different city with people I liked. Anne was willing to go along, and we came very close to moving. But in the end, I decided that if I wanted to re-invent myself, it would be better to try to do that in a place where I had two decades of social capital than to go someplace new where they'd be expecting more of the same and soon would be asking, "What has he done for us lately?"

Shortly before returning from sabbatical, I had lunch with Ann Reichsman, the medical director for my favorite practice in our practice-based research network. Neighborhood Family Practice started out as a small private practice but had grown into a large community health center that is both mission-driven and operationally strong. I thought that doing clinical work there could position me in neutral territory in the wars between the local healthcare systems and could be a good start toward my vague notion of working more at the community-healthcare system interface.

Ann said, "Well, what I really need is a fulltime, female, Spanish-speaking family physician."

O for 3, I thought. *Oh well, at least we'll have a nice lunch together.*

Then, when the curries were almost eaten, she said, "On the other hand, someone always is out sick, or away at a conference, or on parental leave." She paused, and after looking me in the eye, she shook her head, "But you wouldn't want to do that."

"Do what?"

"Be a fill-in doctor."

I thought, *Well, if I want to be open to what comes next, that would give me some slack, and on a platform that is mission-congruent with the direction I want to go.*

Returning from sabbatical, I let my patients know I wouldn't be returning to my university practice, and I did take up part-time at Neighborhood Family Practice as a fill-in doctor on the other side of town. Most of my old patients were gracious about it. Some probably liked their new doctor better and had had a chance to live through the life events together that create a bond. Occasionally, some still call or email me—not for regular care, but when they want to talk with someone who has witnessed them and shared moments that provide understanding or meaning that meets a need at some health or life transition. I harbor some remorse for not keeping up my end of the bargain—for dropping out of the relationship. And I smile at the irony that in order to make more time to study and advocate for making health care more about building relationships than delivering commodities, I am not actually walking the walk. I worry that even as I take on new opportunities to study relationship-centered generalist care, I will have diminished credibility in that work from not actually practicing in the context of ongoing relationships with patients and families.

Returning from sabbatical, my grants were ending, and so I was facing a funding cliff for my academic time. In academic medicine, the coin of the realm is to fund yourself with NIH grants that bring large overhead "indirect cost" payments that support the university (at my school, 60%, on top of the direct costs for doing a project). Back in that environment, I wrote five grant applications, but not for the stealth research I'd gotten good at—proposing a mainstream reductionist project and fitting in the generalist research questions around the edges. Rather, I came out of the reductionist closet and proposed trying to generate new whole-person knowledge from a generalist perspective.

The peer reviews were scathing, and none of these sabbatical-inspired grant applications came anywhere close to being funded. A 24-year-old research assistant made the proper psychological diagnosis—"You know, Kurt, you know how to write applications that get funded. You just don't want to do it anymore."

Ouch. She was right. And I hadn't had the courage to just admit that but felt I had to try to prove something to an impenetrable NIH audience that like everyone, doesn't like someone trying to prove something to them.

The inability to fund my research seemed to seal the end of my academic career. In that failure, and with Anne's support and the sabbatical detachment of being ready to give up almost everything, a vision of a quieter life started emerging. I would ground myself by practicing part-time and working to support community connections. I would move toward a quiet retirement by continuing to try to develop new ways of writing to try to communicate the ancient truths of the generalist healer.

At that moment, I received an email from an old acquaintance, Russ Glasgow, who had just given up his day job to try to shake things up at the National Cancer Institute as their new director of implementation science. On the surface, this looked like an unwelcome tie to what I had run away from with my sabbatical. But the subject line of the email was a friendly, *Do an IPA with me in DC.* Since India Pale Ale was my favorite kind of beer, I said yes, only to find he was inviting me to spend 2 years as a part-time federal employee under the *I*ntergovernmental *P*ersonnel *A*ct. I declined, but when he told me I could do anything I wanted, I decided to call his bluff and ask if I could use the NIH and the larger Department of Health and Human Services (HHS) as a case study to examine the personal and population health effects of boundary spanners—individuals, initiatives, or organizations working across the borders of disciplines or institutions or ways of thinking.

During the sabbatical, the most interesting conversations were with people who were boundary spanners. People often described their boundary-spanning work as the most meaningful and potentially impactful aspect of their lives, but it was also what they were most likely to be maligned for.

So, when Russ said that I could go into the belly of the NIH beast and seek out the boundary spanners and see what they were up to, I said yes. This also provided some cover in my productivity-oriented university environment, as I spent the next 2 years working with him part-time, using the IPA to hatch a new initiative in Promoting Health Across Boundaries (PHAB).

The PHAB initiative started as just a way to have interesting conversations with people who were trying to do boundary-spanning work. This idea did indeed lead to interesting conversations and new relationships with interesting people. At the HHS,

I ended up working on an initiative that pulled together more than a dozen agencies and organizations on a quintessential generalist topic—how to integrate the care of people living with multiple chronic conditions [4].

Back in Cleveland, I tried to set up more interesting PHAB conversations by bringing together a senior faculty member from each of the university's eight schools, plus our county health commissioner [5–7]. When we got together, we could never stay on the agenda because the cross-disciplinary ferment led to so many new ideas. Working to overcome the largely impenetrable challenges of working across inter-school and interdisciplinary boundaries, we taught an innovative interdisciplinary graduate comparative case study course on promoting health across boundaries, and all sorts of small and large spin-off activities in community health and generalism emerged.

Without any particular planning, but just having a general sense of an as yet hazy new direction and being open to emergent opportunities, one thing led to another. One of the PHAB faculty members wanted to apply for a CDC Prevention Research Center, but to be eligible, the institution needs either a public health school or a preventive medicine residency. We had neither, but since I was board certified in preventive medicine and since this seemed congruent with the idea of working more at the healthcare-community health interface, I (reluctantly at the time) agreed to start a residency. Training new physicians to work in the community led to many new connections and opportunities for boundary-spanning work to improve health and equity. The first graduate took over as residency director, and it is now one of only two programs in the country to lead to board eligibility in both preventive medicine and family medicine.

As this was going on in Cleveland, I got a call from someone whose work I'd read but had never met. George Kaplan had done brilliant social epidemiology, including the Alameda County Health and Ways of Living Study. Nearing the usual retirement age, he was cutting loose and pursuing the possibility that computational modeling techniques could allow us to understand how complex systems work and move beyond admiring seemingly intractable problems like inequity, toward actually working together to improve things. This focus on complex systems resonated with how Ben Crabtree and Will Miller had brought complexity science into our work to understand family practice and generalism. But now we had the opportunity to try to understand how inequities emerge over the course of the lifespan of people and societies and what the leverage points might be to make a difference. I felt like a third-grader in a college class but was privileged to join the NIH-funded Network on Complexity, Inequality, and Health (NICH) that he was launching [8].

Since the sabbatical, I had been unwilling to continue the stealth research game of cramming generalist questions into narrow categorical funding boxes, and it had looked like my academic career was in the toilet. But now, ironically, growing from opportunities at the fringes of the NIH, something new was emerging.

The computational modeling collaborators provided by NICH positioned us to be funded for projects in the first two rounds of the new Patient-Centered Outcomes Research Institute. These projects used participatory methods to develop models of how primary care works [9] and how health care that focused on patients' strengths rather than their deficits might be more effective [10]. These projects provided a transition back into the research world, but now focused more on generalist questions and setting up a new way of working collaboratively with communities.

The NICH work also led to a chance conversation with Steve Woolf, who had just become a fellow at the Institute for Integrative Health (now called the Nova Institute) [11]. Steve nominated me to be a fellow as well, to support the still-forming work I wanted to do in community health. The Director, family physician Brian Berman, called me when I was at a weeklong writing workshop, trying to learn a different way of writing creative non-fiction. At the workshop, I realized that I could see parts of the story I wanted to tell next but didn't see a way it could come together. During lunchtime walks at the workshop, a novel formed in my mind. But the voice in the back of my head said—*That's stupid. Who are you to write a novel? You even read more non-fiction than fiction.* The day that Brian called, I'd decided to just get up early every morning to start working on the novel but not to tell anyone I was working on it. Not even Anne. And certainly, not this stranger I was just meeting by phone.

Brian seemed to resonate with supporting the work I was starting to do in community health. But then he asked, "Is there anything else you'd like to do? Anything that's a stretch for you, but that would be personally meaningful, and that you think might make a difference?"

What a great question! I found myself blurting out the whole plot for the novel I'd sworn not to tell anyone about. The upshot was that the Institute supported my time for community health research and development and also supported my time to develop skills as a novelist, which might end up being how I spend my actual retirement, whenever that comes. Subsequently, the Institute has similarly supported the creative work of my colleagues Heidi Gullett and Rebecca Etz. That space to think and act differently has been instrumental in developing new cross-disciplinary work in community health and generalism.

Developmental psychologist Erik Erikson identifies eight stages of development across the lifespan, each with their own tensions. The seventh stage, generativity vs. stagnation, occurs for most people in middle age and involves giving back to society through raising children, work, and community activity. The final stage, integrity vs. despair, occurs during the years when most people retire and involves managing the tensions of letting go of the accomplishments that have stroked our egos and provided our identity, while developing such a solid inward sense of unity and self that it can withstand declining function and eventually letting go of this life.

For these last two stages, serving as a mentor can provide a sense of meaning, generativity, and integrity. I have tried to make that a priority. So many of the resulting relationships start with providing instrumental support for a mentee's career development but end up morphing into being about life and meaning. For me, two mentoring relationships have been particularly generative of emergent directions that build on but transcend the past.

Heidi Gullett joined the faculty a few years after my sabbatical ended. As I tried to help her progress from an outstanding clinician and teacher to an investigator, she showed me a new way of being in partnership with our local community. We used endowment money to support her as the medical school's first population health liaison. Embedded in the county health department, she approached that role to ask, not what she could get, but what she could give. With a community partner and bringing together all the local healthcare systems and health departments, hundreds of organizations, and thousands of individuals, she leads our county's community health improvement plan [12], where the top priority is eliminating structural racism. I started out cashing in some of my local social capital to help with that and related initiatives, but now I am enjoying being just a side player, with Heidi in the lead, in larger initiatives that surpass the work of any one individual or organization. We are swimming against strong currents of greed, anger, and fear, and most days it feels like we are being buffeted backward. But being a small part of something generative and emergent is more meaningful than commanding and controlling something that has little potential to make a real difference.

When the pandemic hit, Heidi served as our county's COVID-19 Incident Commander, and I pivoted my clinical time from family practice to public health practice, following her in efforts to make information, support and testing, and then immunization available to those at highest risk and those being left out by the large healthcare systems.

Starting about the same time as I began working with Heidi, I was also blessed to connect with Rebecca Etz. We'd worked together on a project led by colleagues, and over breakfast she asked for my advice on how, as a cultural anthropologist, she could learn to write in the much more succinct style of the health fields. Having observed how helpful writing retreats were to our colleagues Will Miller and Ben Crabtree, I suggested we try that together. In writing an article together, in sharing our struggles with other things we were trying to communicate, and in talking during walks and meals, we found great commonality in values and mission, but interesting and stimulating differences in background, training, and skills. We realized that those differences could be a great source of creative tension. As we continued to get together for writing retreats, we imagined different ways to try to understand and support generalism and generalist practitioners, and the American Board of Family Medicine Foundation agreed to support our launch of the Larry A. Green Center for the Advancement of Primary Health Care for the Public Good [13].

From the base of the Green Center and from Becca's strong grounding in cultural anthropology, we developed the Person-Centered Primary Care Measure [14, 15] that seeks to radically coopt the current reductionist measurement paradigm by refocusing it on 11 domains—each assessed by a single patient-reported item based on careful analyses of what hundreds of patients, primary care clinicians, and, to a lesser extent, payers, say is important in health care. With Heidi and with support from a Cleveland-area foundation created when a large practice sold itself to one of the local healthcare systems, we launched the Wisdom of Practice Initiative that seeks to discern what generalists are/do that makes a difference in the lives of individuals, families, and communities. And building on 6 years of volunteer board work with the national OCHIN network of community health centers, we are now engaged in two NIH-funded studies to examine how the pandemic has fostered primary care innovations with both positive and negative potential for patients' health and equity, and for the sustainability of the primary care workforce.

At the same time, the platforms on which we were operating were burning. The healthcare systems are increasingly driven by managers who don't understand how to integrate care for whole people and who add administrative burden and unsustainable cost with each patch on the growing fragmentation [16]. Similar forces of fragmentation affect our communities as the commons become smaller and smaller [17].

Starting at the scale of relationships and personal knowing seems like the only viable pathway to help foster the changes needed in our community and healthcare systems. But for a short time, I allowed myself to consider a different, escapist fantasy. I accepted an offer to interview to be the first Bloomberg Distinguished Professor of Primary Care at Johns Hopkins University. At first, I considered the offer only to normalize the idea that this position, at a university without a family medicine department, could be filled by a family physician. But as I spent nearly a year negotiating and expanding the opportunity, it seemed to provide a platform for working toward larger systemic changes.

For the only time in my career, I let my boss (the dean) know I was looking elsewhere. She asked what I'd really like to do. We talked about how the local environment was looking less and less supportive for family medicine and primary care, and how a new platform was needed to support this and our emerging work in community health and equity. She listened and worked to support an emerging vision. As a result, I turned down the Hopkins offer and launched the Center for Community Health Integration [18], which functions as a boundary-spanning basic science department at the medical school. The CHI Center is about *research and development for community health and integrated, personalized care*, and we are working to make it a platform for developing the next generation of boundary spanners to advance community health, equity, and generalism. It provides a platform for doing meaningful work and for mentoring the next generation. But it adds back even more of the administrative and fundraising responsibilities that I'd tried to shed, and I'm once again starting to feel the fragmenting pulls of doing too many things.

What is different now is the detachment from the outcomes, an increasing focus on the next generation, and while supporting the community health work, putting most of my energy back into my roots in working to bring to light the treasures of generalism that feel like they are being lost.

Recruiting and engaging new people, working with Heidi and Becca, and trying to support their careers and lives, seeing how they are better than me in so many areas of this work, has rejuvenated me in focusing on what is meaningful, difficult, and under-supported, and it gives me hope that the work will continue when I do finally retire. It is liberating to be at the life stage where I don't have to prove anything to anyone, to be able to approach work and life in a more joyful and hopefully more selfless way, and to pursue things that on the surface appear to be bad career and life moves, but that might make a difference and that actually help to sand off the rough edges keeping me selfish and separate.

Preparing to Let Go

Recently, I visited two friends for a long weekend. In the Sunday morning conversation over breakfast, I started a sentence, "If I could control my own destiny, I'd...."

Geri deGruy interrupted, "Who says you can't control your own destiny?"

"OK, you're right, Geri. But it sounds arrogant to say I can control my own destiny."

I paused and started over, "For the portion of my destiny for which I might have some agency.... what I was going to say is—I'd like to take another sabbatical."

Geri's husband Frank piled on, "Well why can't you? You're a grown-assed man."

Point taken. So, 15 years after the first one, I started planning another sabbatical. When you do that as you approach 65 years old, people think you are going to retire. So, as with the first sabbatical, I needed a story to tell others since, to some extent, that frames the external opportunities. But the real focus is the internal story since that's the only part of my own destiny for which I really can have any control.

The purpose of this sabbatical, like the first one, would be to refocus on what is most important. But this time, the internal and external stories need to be more aligned. Rather than disengaging to create space to figure out what's next, I'll need to unify effort around a few interrelated projects that all relate to understanding how generalism works. It seems to me that many of the things that have been done on a policy level to try to improve generalism and primary care haven't really understood what is special and valuable about it, and as a result, many have actually made things worse—more fragmented and more impersonal.

In this second sabbatical, I would let a lot of projects go that don't really need me anymore. I'd continue to support my colleagues at the CHI Center and others that I'm mentoring but devote more energy to working with others to advance understanding of how to integrate and personalize care for whole people. And I'd resume getting up early every morning to complete the final revision of the novel.

This time of stepping away from usual activities would be a chance to let my junior colleagues spread their wings in leadership, for which they are both ready and better suited than I.

I discussed this sabbatical plan with CHI Center Associate Director Heidi Gullett and Executive Director Jim Bindas, and they generously agreed to support it. When I talked about the plan with my Green Center Co-director, Rebecca Etz, I thought she'd be delighted. She wasn't. She listened, then challenged me, "You don't want to make a change for a year. You want to make a change for the next five to ten years."

It's good to have friends who can listen and then tell you what you really mean.

So now we're in the process of proposing Heidi to take over as CHI Center Director, with me moving to a behind the scenes mentoring role. We'll see what happens.

Anne, who is a year older than me, retired a few months ago from her work as a pathologist. Recalling how helpful it was to recommit to the relationship when I took my sabbatical at our empty nester transition, I decided to do the same at this new life stage. An opportunity came sooner than planned when she suffered a severe ankle injury in a biking accident that required surgery and 2 months of non-weight bearing. Being in the caregiver role was both gratifying and a sobering foreshadowing of what might be ahead for both of us. She's starting to walk again, and we're both benefiting from a physical therapist who helps us to train our bodies. But we're looking at moving to a single-story house that will be better for aging in place, as we transition to discover together what it means to have one of us retired and one working but with the striving for the detachment from outcomes, and from self, that is necessary to truly love. Or maybe that's how both of us will be approaching life. We have a new grandchild, and I'm looking for personal ways to be part of his life, even as I try to find ways to make some small contribution to improving the world into which he will grow.

This life stage and career change, even more than the sabbatical, is helping me prepare for the ultimate letting go. Death is closer now. The major work of this transition is to get over my small self and to deeply experience and participate in the unity of life. I will try to use these coming years (if I am blessed with years) to advance my detachment from self even as I work to strengthen loving connections. I'll work to advance my spiritual practice and use the resulting energy to give back to the world, even as I get ready to leave it. I'll try to approach each minute with the recognition that my householder's life is merely a platform for a spiritual practice that is my best chance to leave things a bit better than I found them.

This practice is the hardest thing I've ever attempted, and I've been working on it for two decades with painfully slow progress but growing longing. Guided by an enlightened teacher, the practice is an 8-point program [19, 20] that involves: meditating twice a day, using a mantram to focus the mind during the day and night, slowing down and setting priorities, working to develop one-pointed attention, working to overcome conditioned habits, putting others first, and engaging in spiritual fellowship and reading.

I am an introvert. But rather than approaching this next life phase with reticence and shyness, I'll try openness and humility. I'll try to carry forward some of the lessons from the sabbatical while learning new ones. My father's bowl and Larry's email remain prominently displayed in my office. But it's still hard for me to imagine actually retiring. The work that I see on the horizon still looks like a better platform than retirement for my unrealized aspirations of selfless service, relationships, and connection with the Unity of life.

When the time does come to step away for good, I hope to be ready to:

> balance action with reflection,
>> invest in old and new relationships,
>> take time to create space for new learning and meaning,
>> detach from the outcomes of actions,
>> be open to emergence in the face of uncertainty, and,
>> prepare to let go of myself so I can be drawn into our oneness.

References

1. Stange KC, Jaén CR, Flocke SA, Miller WL, Crabtree BF, Zyzanski SJ. The value of a family physician. J Fam Pract. 1998;46(5):363–8.
2. Blue Mountain Journal. Detachment: learning to live in freedom. Tomales, California: Blue Mountain Center for Meditation; 2023. https://www.bmcm.org/inspiration/journals/.
3. Stange KC. The generalist approach. Ann Fam Med. 2009;7(3):198–203.
4. Bayliss EA, Bonds DE, Boyd CM, Davis MM, Finke B, Fox MH, et al. Understanding the context of health for persons with multiple chronic conditions: moving from what is the matter to what matters. Ann Fam Med. 2014;12(3):260–9.
5. Promoting Health Across Boundaries (PHAB). Promoting Health Across Boundaries https://case.edu/medicine/phab/.
6. PHAB Staff and Writing Committee, Aungst H, Ruhe M, Stange KC, PHAB Cleveland Advisory Committee, Allan TM, et al. Boundary spanning and health: invitation to a learning community. London J Prim Care. 2012;4(2):109–15.
7. Stange KC. Refocusing knowledge generation, application and education: raising our gaze to promote health across boundaries. Am J Prev Med. 2011;41(4 Suppl 3):S164–S9.
8. Kaplan GA, Diez Roux AV, Simon CP, Galea S. Growing inequality: bridging complex systems, population health, and health disparities. Washington, DC: Westphalia Press; 2017. p. 332.
9. Homa L, Rose J, Hovmand PS, Cherng ST, Riolo RL, Kraus A, et al. A participatory model of the paradox of primary care. Ann Fam Med. 2015;13(5):456–65.
10. Aungst H, Baker M, Bouyer C, Catalano B, Cintron M, Cohen NB, et al. Identifying personal strengths to help patients manage chronic illness. Washington, DC: Patient-Centered Outcomes Research Institute (PCORI); 2019.
11. Nova Institute. Transforming Health. https://novainstituteforhealth.org/
12. HIP-Cuyahoga. HIP-Cuyahoga. https://hipcuyahoga.org/.
13. Green Center. Larry A. Green Center for the Advancement of Primary Health Care for the Public Good. https://www.green-center.org/
14. Larry A. Green Center for the Advancement of Primary Health Care for the Public Good. Person-Centered Primary Care Measure. https://www.green-center.org/pcpcm.
15. Etz RS, Zyzanski SJ, Gonzalez MM, Reves SR, O'Neal JP, Stange KC. A new comprehensive measure of high-value aspects of primary care. Ann Fam Med. 2019;17(3):221–30.
16. Tarn DM, Wenger NS, Stange KC. Small solutions for primary care are part of a larger problem. Ann Intern Med. 2022;175(8):1179–80. https://www.ncbi.nlm.nih.gov/pubmed/35759763.
17. Stange KC. The problem of fragmentation and the need for integrative solutions. Ann Fam Med. 2009;7(2):100–3.
18. CHI Center. Center for Community Health Integration. https://case.edu/medicine/healthintegration/.
19. Easwaran E. Passage meditation: a complete spiritual practice. Tomales, CA: Nilgiri Press; 2016.
20. Blue Mountain Center for Meditation. The eight-point program of passage meditation. https://www.bmcm.org/learn/eight-point/.

Chapter 11
When God Gives You a Good Kick in Your Rear End

Tochi Iroku-Malize

Editors' Introduction
Born in the U.S. to Nigerian immigrant parents, a surgeon, and a midwife, Tochi Iroku-Malize knew from childhood that she wanted to be a doctor, despite the prejudice she describes in elementary school. After her father spent a year volunteering in Nigeria doing surgery when Tochi was in high school, he invited the whole family to go live in Nigeria, an experience that shaped Tochi's view of the world and where she went to college and medical school. As a native-born U.S. citizen, and also an international medical graduate, the child of immigrants who made sure that their offspring had the best education, Tochi had the opportunity to see the world from a variety of viewpoints and cultures. She knew that what healthcare was available and appropriate for a person or a family depended very much on where they came from and where and how they lived. She formalized that knowledge with an MPH in Health Policy & Management. She went on to rise to the top in every site where she worked in the educational, clinical, and administrative worlds, including the Presidency of the American Academy of Family Physicians in 2022–2023. On the way, she learned that being unstoppable requires choices and setting priorities. The spirit was willing, but the body had its own vulnerabilities. Tochi emerged from an illness more connected to her relationships with family and friends and better able to put limits on her other commitments. A tough challenge for one with so many talents. Yet she succeeds!

There is nothing like God giving you a good kick in your rear end to get you going in the right direction.

That is how I look at the turn of events that led to me changing my perspective on leadership, career aspirations and goals.

T. Iroku-Malize (✉)
Zucker School of Medicine at Hofsta/Northwell, Hempstead, NY, USA
e-mail: tmalize@northwell.edu; Mmassot@northwell.edu

I had done the usual things needed to move along the trajectory of academic medicine, which, to be honest, was not my original plan. I was going to do international medicine and save the world. I digress.

Let's start a few decades ago. I was born in Brooklyn, N.Y., to immigrant parents, one a medical student and the other a nurse midwife. We lived in a small apartment, a railroad apartment, where the bathroom at the end of the hall was shared by others. I can still remember the green Formica table in the main eating area/kitchen. My dad had a scholarship from his country of origin, Nigeria, but once the Biafran War began, all Nigerian students were told to choose a side, and he sided with the people of his ethnicity, the Igbos. So goodbye scholarship, hello mom working two jobs to help with the stipend he received for working in the labs. Medical school was not cheap then as it is not at present.

Eventually, he would graduate from medical school and complete his surgical residency. We would move to an urban area in New Jersey, and my mom would get her nursing degree (all the while working two jobs and now raising four kids). My first gift that I wished for was a Fisher Price doctor's kit. I loved spinning the thermometer and using the sphygmomanometer (say that three times fast), the reflex hammer, and the stethoscope. All in the wonderful primary colors of red, yellow, and blue.

In elementary school, I excelled in all subjects as I listened to the mantra, "You must get a great education, you cannot waste your brain cells." So I was usually at the top of my class for every subject. When we moved to the suburbs, white house, black trim, pool in the backyard, Cadillac in the driveway, I guess you could say we had finally made it. In my new school, I was one of a few black students, and the administrators refused to put me in my usual gifted class section. They stated that my "A's" at my previous school (a black neighborhood) were not equivalent to the "A's" in their school. They actually put me in a remediation class on my first day. My mom marched in the next day and told them she would not sign the paperwork for me to be put into that class but rather that I should be placed in a regular classroom and given a chance to prove myself. Within a week, I was moved from one section to another untill I was finally in the gifted section. I would eventually be among a few who were taken to the high school for special math classes.

A counselor once came to our school to do an evaluation on our future careers. And as I had mentioned previously, I always knew I would be a doctor. So I filled out my form and wrote in "doctor." The next day, the evaluations were returned to us, and my result was that I would be a "secretary." I informed the counselor that he had made a mistake on my form as I was going to be a doctor. He politely patted my head and said, "Oh no, you cannot be a doctor, but if you work hard enough, one day you can be a secretary in a doctor's office." My mom was really pissed when I let her know about this after school and warned me sternly that I should never, ever, ever let anyone define who I am.

Fast forward decades later, I did become a doctor and became a family medicine resident.

As a resident, I was always looking for methods to make learning and teaching more accessible to those involved. I did not believe in the rote memorization of facts

11 When God Gives You a Good Kick in Your Rear End

that sometimes plagued medical education. I liked the idea of using various methods to learn—auditory, visual, tactile. or a combination of those. So when I became chief resident and was in charge of creating the didactic curriculum and schedule for my fellow residents, I was excited to create something new. Key skills were needed to be able to negotiate with community physicians and with specialists outside of family medicine to make themselves available to our program (without pay) for topics that they usually did not provide. This worked out well and led to my being offered a continuous role in residency education upon graduation.

As the new lead for hospital medicine, a specialty that had just evolved as I was leaving residency, I once again created opportunities for residents to learn new material in different ways, but I also found myself having to create faculty development sessions for my hospitalists, to whom I had assigned rotations on the teaching service. Lucky for me, a new simulation lab had just opened up, and I was the first to sign up physicians to use the facility. A great way to check the application of knowledge learned in the regular settings. I spent many days, nights, weekends, and holidays honing my academic craft. I traveled to innumerable academic conferences, learning everything there was to know about undergraduate, graduate, and continuing medical education. I took lessons from local, national, and international peers and reformatted them to work within our institution. Before you knew it, I was presenting at these same venues.

Eventually I was offered an associate family medicine program director role while still director of the hospitalist program, and I continued to push for research and scholarly activity. If we didn't have a champion in a particular area, I would step in and do the work until I could train someone to lead the cause. Creating a new innovative home visit curriculum? No worries. Goodbye Saturdays. Revamping nursing home curriculum? Who needs Sundays? Not to mention the operational sides of academic medicine along with operational clinical medicine and its regulations, policies, procedures, privileging, accreditation, reviews, budgets, human resources, risk mitigation, and on and on. So long weeknights.

My efforts did not go unnoticed. I did enjoy my job. It was ever changing and engaging, and I was able to utilize my creative juices to implement projects and programs that started as mere ideas. My saying was that "Nothing is impossible," and fortunately I worked in an organization that was ever expanding and also very innovative. So, I was left to my own devices to do what was needed to move us forward academically and clinically. As long as the work was done and the financial margin stayed positive, no worries.

Then came the announcement that a new medical school would be formed. I was tagged to join the group of academics within the organization to help create the new curriculum. This was a collective group of individuals from all clinical specialties as well as from academia, and it was phenomenal. The meetings were held early in the morning because we all still had to do our day job. Goodbye sleep. But what eventually came forth was the creation of a truly innovative method of training medical students. During this process, I learned that Family Medicine was not going to be a department within the medical school but rather a subdivision of Medicine. Stop the presses!

Now I had to advocate for the creation of a family medicine department in this new medical school. Sidebar—I had been doing advocacy work since I was a resident. My program director, Dr. Richard Bonanno, had gotten me involved in the New York State Academy of Family Physicians (NYSAFP) and the American Academy of Family Physicians (AAFP). And I had become the resident representative for the state and would eventually do advocacy work on behalf of family medicine and our communities in Albany and Washington, DC. Stating my case in front of legislators and their aides had become second nature, and I was well prepared to do so within my organization. My advocacy experience helped me successfully present the advantages of family medicine being its own department in the medical school, which led to the creation of the department, not only for the school but also for the tertiary sites within the health system that did not have family medicine departments.

By this point, I had become the chair of family medicine for both the school and the health system, with its numerous hospitals and ambulatory sites. I was working triple time to advance academics and the clinical operations and projects for my family medicine colleagues. There was still a lot of pushback from the other primary care specialties, as they were not keen on family medicine actually encroaching on their territory. Mind you, when I was able to pull the data on just how many family physicians were in our system, a lot of people had to lift their jaws off the floor. These physicians had all along been listed under internal medicine.

I'd be remiss if I didn't speak a bit about the relationships I had with my colleagues and mentors as I moved along in my career. Since residency, I had a close-knit group of residents across all 3 years. We were of similar ages, and a number of us expanded our families along the same timeline. In fact, there are three of us who were pregnant at the same time and had our children attend the same schools until they went to high school and then college. We continue to share our hopes and dreams to this day. In fact, the three of us would be together in a hospital room in New York City in 2019.

There was Dr. Bonanno, already mentioned, as my program director. I would go to him for advice as needed while a resident, then as a faculty member, and eventually as his associate program director. He was stern but very open hearted. And I would only discover how much work he provided to the community outside of business hours when I took over his role as program director and members of the community-based organizations reached out to me to schedule the regular activities he had been involved in. He is a true servant leader, and I was even more impressed and inspired to do the same. I trusted his opinion implicitly, as well as that of my former associate program director, Dr. Scott Kirsch. In fact, when I became program director, I would later hire them as my faculty. So much for retirement! And these two gentlemen were the ones I turned to for advice about whether I should take the position as inaugural chair for the new medical school.

Setting new goals, creating steps to implement them, and strategizing on the best ways to advance the mission of family medicine became my daily work. Saying "Yes" to multiple non-mission-based assignments and projects in order to play nicely in the sandbox was my default. I allowed others to "borrow" my ideas and present them as their own by saying to myself that it was for the greater good and that it did not matter if I was not given credit. Watching others quickly advance up the ladder in the organization from both the academic and corporate lanes while I toiled feverishly and humbly became my norm. At the end of each academic year, I would tell myself that it was time to make a change, do something different, claim my prize? 1 year turned to three, then five, then seven, and before I knew it, I had been doing this for 10 years! My family would tell me to make a change. But I continued, out of loyalty and out of the realization that if not me, then who? Because I was the only clinical chair that looked like me in the whole organization. Those who were up and coming needed to see someone in a leadership position that they could aspire to reach.

I had done as I had seen being done by my mentors. I took on mentees from within and outside family medicine and medicine itself. I believed that it was my duty to give constructive criticism with options for improvement to anyone who asked for my help. Some would take the advice, and others did not. As long as I was fair and true in the information I was sharing, I felt I was doing the right thing. I did get validation on occasion. There was a particularly trying morning at the administrative office of my clinical site. It was truly stressful. And then I received a phone call from a former resident who was practicing in another state. They called just to tell me thank you—paraphrasing here – "Thank you so much Dr. Iroku! I just saw a patient and remembered one of the sessions you taught and it was exactly what I needed to do for them! It was great!" So, my less than stellar morning took on a new light, and I was good to go for the rest of the day.

This would work for different moments along my path, but all the while, I would get little signs that I should change my process. Things would go wrong. Little ones, then bigger ones. Naysayers and backstabbers (yes, we all know they exist) would siderail projects or try to sully my reputation. But I would take the high road and let it go while continuing to work hard. 7 days a week, almost 18-hour days.

Then God kicked me where the sun don't shine. I was feeling ill. Everyone thought I was overworked. I went to my family physician in the spring of 2019. Told her to do all the tests, lab work, radiological studies, EKG, because something wasn't right. And lo and behold, I was correct.

I had a life-threatening illness and ended up being hospitalized for four out of 6 months. I ended up having my skull opened three times, going to rehab once, being intubated twice, and dropping down to 113 lbs. (with my 5′ 11″ frame).

Suddenly, I was delegating my workload to six different people. When I was able, I would give input from the hospital bed or from home. My new goal was to stay alive. At this point, my relationships turned to my family. My siblings were my tightest group, followed by my nuclear family, my mom, my maternal uncle, and my best friend. For work relationships, I didn't want to burden them with my daily struggles. I knew they were worried, and it was better to only give them positive information. Besides, it would not help them to fall apart while carrying on with the work required of our department and service line. Patients still needed to be cared for, budgets still needed to be completed, educational sessions still needed to be presented.

I can say that my family relies on our religious faith, and there were numerous prayer circles happening across the globe. This was important in addition to the medical science that was the mainstay of my treatment. I can also say that my core medical team showed such empathy that I felt validated for my approach to my own patients. Even with a medical degree, when you are laying in a stretcher or hospital bed with flimsy gowns and odd-shaped, uncomfortable mattresses, listening to a lot of jargon about how your body is responding, or not, to treatment, it is nice to have an empathetic individual relaying the information.

By January 2020, I was working slowly. My meetings had been reduced and my prior projects were being run by others. March 2020 brought COVID which worked for me because administrators and execs now did everything virtually. I was not able to see patients till the summer of 2020 (hooking myself up to a TPN bag at night while I slept to keep my weight from falling further). I look back at the pictures of myself at that time with my PPE (personal protective equipment) and just marvel at the skeleton frame trying to care for others.

By the time the fall came, I was no longer as tolerant of bullshit (BS) as I had been before.

I had learned to say "No" while ill. As I recovered, I realized my top priority was being alive for at least the next 5 years. So "No" if it did not fulfill my personal mission of creating an environment for people to thrive, live healthy, and be their best self. "No" if it was going to interfere with the quality time I had designated to spending with my family. My kids were now older (two in college and one about to start college). "No" if it was going to prevent me from having my own space to think and reflect with a cup of tea and a good book while sitting outside!

I had also learned to speak up more forcefully. If I saw something that wasn't kosher, I would say it. In a nice tone, but firmly. And if I spoke up and was ignored, I would repeat myself. Because my illness taught me that I had nothing to lose but my life, and that I only had one life, so I'd better make the best use of it. Otherwise, I was wasting my time.

So, I have been bolder and have dropped certain projects and taken on others. Ditto with relationships. Be it with family, friends, peers, or patients. With family, I learned to be a bit more patient and to make sure they understood how important they are to me on a daily basis. Because, let's be honest, no one really knows when our last interaction will be. I have always been quick to forgive and to squash a disagreement or argument. I am now more measured in my responses and more tolerant of mistakes.

In terms of friends, I have taken the advice I give to others. Reach out and find a way to socialize. Even if it is by having a virtual lunch or dinner. Having a beverage and meal and chatting away on Zoom does wonders for the soul. It is great to laugh wholeheartedly and then just climb the stairs to your bedroom after the event is over. This worked with my close friends from medical school. We are all in different states or countries, but we were able to have frank conversations about everything that has happened in our lives over the past 25 years. For the first time, the four of us met together for a mini-vacation in Europe, a girls' extended weekend. Just in time for my birthday. No hubbies, no kids. And then, of course, there is my current best friend, also a family doctor, who was in my N.Y. hospital setting up decorations for me when I was first admitted to the oncology suite to begin chemotherapy and later saved my life during the annual congress and conference for family medicine held in Pennsylvania, which we were both attending. I had been complaining of a headache, and she was able to get me to the local hospital, where I was diagnosed with a cerebral hemorrhage. Prior to this, we would communicate maybe every other week. Now we can chat (audio, video, or text) daily, regardless of where either of us is located. She is now an official member of my family. Shout out to you, Debo! We try to hold each other accountable in terms of having a personal life outside of work.

With peers and patients, I have tried to take a little more time to be empathetic. But not to the detriment of my own wellbeing. Whatever I can do to assist them in their own journeys, I will do. I have learned to accept empathy as well. It is no longer important to be the superwoman in all spaces to all people. I am willing to admit when I am feeling tired and when I just cannot take on another thing. And I am willing to accept compliments and criticism. Being tolerant of varying perceptions and belief systems with regard to health, politics, etc., is a daily process in which I am willing to engage. However, I do it in an honest fashion. As mentioned before, I have cut the BS out of my life on a large scale.

Then there is the relationship I have with myself. I have learned to be more kind and forgiving. I understand now that I cannot be all things to all people and that I will never be perfect. I reflect yearly, quarterly, monthly, and weekly on my goals and strategies to get there. If an activity is not aligned, it gets a hard pass.

I know my time—daily and here on earth—is precious.

I love what I do, and I still work hard (but smart), so I will continue on the path towards making sure others who see me understand that they too can reach their goal and hopefully not bow to the external pressures to deplete who they are. A number of people have passed through my sphere of influence who have given me feedback that they have taken notes, here and there, and applied it to their own lives. With success.

Which means I must be doing something right.

Chapter 12
Leaving My Patients, Losing Myself

Cynthia G. Carmichael

Editors' Introduction

Dr. Cynthia Carmichael and her brother, Dr. Kevin Carmichael, began treating HIV patients in Miami in the early 1990s during their family medicine residency. At that time, HIV was the province of the infectious disease specialists, but the population of people needing HIV care in Miami—Haitian immigrants, intravenous drug users, and MSM (men who have sex with men)—was much larger and needier than the specialists could handle. Cynthia and Kevin Carmichael wrote a primary care textbook on HIV, HIV/AIDS Primary Care Handbook, together with an HIV specialist, to spread the word to other family doctors around the country. Cynthia Carmichael went on to practice in neighborhood health centers in the Bay Area, where she continued her commitment to underserved populations and HIV patients, now with more options like group visits but still with many challenges. Later, she joined the Kaiser Permanente Practice in Richmond, where resources were more abundant, and some of her patients followed. There, she won the 2017 Teaching Award for Excellence in Clinical Medical Education. With a strong family history of Alzheimer's dementia and familiarity with her father Lynn's unremitting downward course, she was alert to the initial issues for herself before anyone else. The loss of her father's family medicine wisdom and his anchoring role in their family was a deep sadness not only for her but also for broader family medicine as well. Lynn Carmichael MD was one of the founders of family medicine as a discipline in the U.S. who convinced the general practitioners of the late 1960s that Family Medicine needed to be birthed as a specialty. Cynthia carried on his legacy in California in family medicine and will be teaching all who know her about grace in the face of calamity.

C. G. Carmichael (✉)
Formerly Family Physician at Campus Shared Services, University of California at Berkeley, Berkeley, CA, USA

One day, as I was getting ready to drive to the community clinic to precept the new interns, my husband said, "Something is not right with you!"

I immediately responded, "Do you think it is Alzheimer's?" I asked that as my father, my paternal grandfather, my paternal aunt, and a cousin all died from Alzheimer's dementia.

I went to work that morning but felt insecure, and that was the last time I went back to the clinic. Shortly thereafter, I resigned from my student health position at UC Berkeley and asked a colleague to take on those HIV-positive students that I had cared for.

Then I went home, and my husband and I cried because I knew I could not go back to medicine in case I become confused or missed a diagnosis. Once the diagnosis of Alzheimer's was given to me, I found myself remembering the details of how my father deteriorated and was ultimately unable to speak clearly. Furthermore, the disease comes along with a terminal diagnosis.

My disease is early for now, but I worry about losing my speech and possibly my continence. My days are filled with reading and writing, thank goodness. And I appreciate my friends who love me and visit regularly.

My husband is my caregiver and is kind, patient, and loving. I am afraid of my future, but I also fear for our daughters, who are both in their early 30s. They too are at risk for Alzheimer's.

I wrote some time ago about losing my father and how I now realize that our parents enabled my brothers and me to continue our lives without really dealing with the ugly realities of his dementia. We went on our way, my youngest brother, an elite bicycle racer, and my older brother a family physician in Tucson. And I, perhaps closest to my father, completed my family medicine residency at the program he had founded at Jackson Memorial Hospital in Miami, Florida, and then settled with our young family in Berkeley, CA.

I have ambivalent feelings about the choices my parents made, though I don't blame them for their wishes. I wish I would have been with my parents the whole time of his dementia, as we loved him so much, but that was not to be.

Last week, I found an old journal of my deceased mother. She wrote: "Our marriage has changed; I don't like him, he pays me no attention …. I feel so sorry for him and I pray I do not suffer his fate …. I don't think he even recognizes me anymore." In another entry in her journal, she wrote that she had wanted them both to come live with us in Berkeley. But by that time, she had had a stroke and died not long after. So many tragedies from this disease. Here are two poems I wrote about my parents:

1. ***A Walk with my Father:*** *Much is the same as always; an early departure, half-hearted complaints about my mother. The occasional pause as you collect the refuse we pass along the way. But some things have changed—your frame, slighter next to mine, your "Popeye" calves diminished. And you lose words, whole memories. I can see them slip away, I hold my breath, watch your face. Gone is Osprey, the beautiful bird, whose silhouette you taught me to know. Gone, the name of your son. Your train of thought moves on without you. On the platform, your hollow body stands beside ours. Waiting.*
2. *When I was a child my mother sang in the kitchen. She no longer remembers the songs she sang. Nor can I, but I know she hummed when she forgot the words or changed tunes*

without skipping a beat. The songs make me cry so I have to pause again and again to keep my voice steady. My mother mouths the words. She remembers! she hums! she sings! and by the time that We Shall Over Come comes around again we are singing out loud together. We'll walk hand and hand.

I do believe we are singing together, my father 4 years dead, We are singing, deep in my heart, We are singing, We are not Afraid.

As we got older, my two brothers and I feared for years about the prospect of one or more of us inheriting our father's Alzheimer's disease. I know my father was afraid. I think I knew deep inside for years that it would be me to follow in my father's footsteps to dementia. I know now that I inherited his disease just as my father's paternal grandfather inherited his Alzheimer's, just as I knew then that at some point, I would follow in the tragic footsteps of my father as he traversed the country of Alzheimer's and modeled acceptance of this horrible disease. Toward the end of his life, I listened to him as he repeated again and again, "I know it is hard for your mother, but I am not unhappy."

I struggle to accept this disease—I rage against it daily, and I am not alone. Heredity is destiny now, but soon that will not be the case. We have the means to edit problematic genes like those that are associated with Alzheimer's and sickle cell disease, and more, perhaps, though not quite yet. Of course, our daughters are aware of my disease, and they will avail themselves of those methods to prevent such horrible losses as my father and now, potentially, Me!

My Medical Career

I enjoyed my family medicine residency in South Florida; the community was quite poor, and I loved my patients. I had a young woman who wanted to get pregnant, and she was a "dog person," like me. She had no interest in laboring in a hospital. She said, "I've watched so many dogs give birth! I can do it myself." I tried to dissuade her, but in the end, she was fine, and she delivered her own baby with her mother's help.

I had another patient who had intractable hiccups. This was early when HIV was just beginning to ravage our community. At endoscopy, the diagnosis was severe thrush, and he was treated appropriately and recovered, although HIV took his life. At that time, the only medication available was AZT, which was not very efficacious, and the loss of life was horrific. In that community, I became a family doctor like my dad. I emulated him as I had learned so much from him, and I still remembered and utilized so many of his 'pearls' in my own practice—until now.

Since 1997, I have practiced in North Richmond, California, in a community that is mostly African American and Hispanic. Later, I would work at Kaiser Permanente, less than a mile from my old clinic. My father would have admired Kaiser's "constituency-based model," although he would have added "Person-centered Health Care."

I practiced in a community where crack cocaine was rampant. Despite that, I loved walking across the street to check on my patients, and they were always grateful. I remember when the teenager across the street came to the clinic with a loaded gun! We talked a lot, but he continued to play with guns. He wanted to see how it felt. The clinic was monitored daily by the police. He was a menace, and his single mother was overwhelmed with her life and her children's behavior. He was murdered. I still wonder now how I could have helped him.

It was also the time of HIV, and many of my patients died. Understandably, a few patients were suspicious about being experimented on, like the subjects in the Tuskegee Experiment. Some people refused to take the pills. Over the years, I started a monthly luncheon with our HIV+ patients to discuss their questions of all kinds. I was delighted and gratified that a lot of my patients and others attended. When one patient was reluctant to attend the group, other participants urged him and others to attend. We even wrote a poem for him. Each participant spoke of their own volition, and it was moving to hear what came out. I still have the final draft of their spoken words:

> *Tony's happiness makes me happy.*
> *He came to the breakfast happy and full of glee.*
> *I knew him when he was sad and blue.*
> *He came to the breakfast happy and full of glee,*
> *Even though his dreams are very crazy, he gets up every morning.*
> *He was so sick just a few weeks ago*
> *And now his face is full of glow.*
> *I love the gift of life, It goes day by day.*
> *Tony shares it with his friends and daughter*
> *And touches others along the way* [1]

Once I made a home visit to a patient who I suspected was not taking his antiretroviral medicines. When he opened the door, I saw that he had plastic boxes full of antiretroviral medicines from the floor to the ceiling. With a lot of counseling and discussion about the importance of taking antiretroviral medicine daily, some patients became more vigilant about taking their medicines, which encouraged other patients to try what their doctor and friends recommended.

I am so lucky to have become close to my patients over the years. I am in touch with many of them as we have become friends now that I am no longer practicing.

I wrote this piece after I started practicing in North Richmond, CA, in my first job 1997. It remains my most cherished practice.

> **What I Love about my practice:** *Driving to work, I love the juxtaposition between the oil refineries, the crisscross of railroad tracks ... and then the suddenly newly constructed single-family homes, little and not so little boxes on the hillside ... and then turning the corner, watching the rooster named Big Red cross the street. And my patient, Mr. H, walking in the middle of the street in his blue jumpsuit, wearing the latex gloves I gave him from the clinic, straining against his overloaded shopping cart full of recycling. I love the groups of men standing on the corner ... the churches, empty in the morning, sometimes full in the afternoon, when well-dressed people mourn their losses and the hearse awaits.*
>
> *Being at work, I love arriving early and opening the window shades and looking out and letting the sun in. A few minutes of solace before the storm.*

12 Leaving My Patients, Losing Myself

I love closing the door behind me and being alone with my patient, leaving the world behind, and entering, contemplating, observing, recognizing, respecting, puzzling over, touching, another person, another Life. I can ask after the children, inquire about the swollen knee, the painful ear, the murdered niece, the many murdered nephews, the headache, the heart ache.

I get to laugh and cry, sometimes in close proximity to each other. I get to feel the firm gravid belly, and the chubby toddler thighs, and the lump that shouldn't be here or there.

I get to lance the abscess and ignore the familiar stench.

I have to deliver the bad news about the HIV test, or the lump that should not be there. I have to say no to refilling the narcotic prescription that somehow got lost, or stolen, or eaten by the dog, or fell into the toilet, or in a puddle, or blown away, or left on the bus, or all of the above.

I have to bear witness to the ravages of heroin and crack, of guns, of homelessness, of hopelessness, of self-worthlessness ... every single day.

Leaving work, I love knowing that the clinic was built on the site of a popular blues club. A patient once remarked that it seemed appropriate that we should be here, trying to save lives, on the same ground where blood was often spilled during fights at Minnie Lou's place ... a rough neighborhood.

I love closing the window shades and humming a few bars of the blues and knowing I will be back tomorrow.

After many years at North Richmond, a colleague recruited me for Kaiser Permanente. I was unhappy about losing my patients but intrigued by what I had heard about Kaiser and my father's high opinion of it. When I left North Richmond, I cried daily, missing my patients so much. As it turned out, many of my patients at North Richmond came with me to Kaiser, which pleased me immensely.

My husband noted years ago that what I really love about my patients is listening about their lives, their loves, and how they get through their day. Such joy it is to learn about someone, to touch their bodies, and to reveal their illness, their loss, and their laughter. I try to "Recognize every patient." I want that for myself, my children, and my friends. What a gift—I hope it is reciprocated.

I learned a lot working at Kaiser. I liked that my patients could go to several Kaiser pharmacies in the building. I liked that I could do house calls as I did when I was at North Richmond. I liked that I could pick up the phone at any time to speak with a specialist if I had concerns about a particular patient matter or diagnosis. I liked the weekly sessions with my colleagues learning about the latest changes in Kaiser protocols. It was a demanding job with the hours of work I did at home both in the evening and in the morning before work. I viewed the next day's patient diagnoses and made occasional phone calls to check in with patients. I liked that I was reminded about specific patient details—a smoker, say, with reminder to refer for lung cancer screening, or a person living with HIV. I as well liked that each patient had a continuity physician and also that if the patient did not like their doctor, they could just call Kaiser and find another doctor.

As much as I admired working at Kaiser, some patients have reported that their doctors don't look at them at all; they just look at the computer! That makes me feel sad as my encounters with patients have so often given me joy and laughter, and I have loved learning more about my patients. What a gift!

I am a poet and many of my poems reflect my experience with patients. These poems reflect some of what I have learned about my patients and about myself.

1. *The toenails I clip ricochet off the walls and ceiling. Sometimes I use both hands to wield the heavy-duty nail shears. Oh how tongues loosen and what stories emerge when patients rest their feet in my lap, when I adjust my glasses and set to trimming! From my father I learned to hold the hand of my patient when counting the pulse, to gently hold the arm against my body when measuring the blood pressure. Then I understood the privilege of touching and listening, of squeezing pimples and cutting toenails, especially for elders who cannot always reach their own toenails to clip.*
2. *At some point it was clear that he was not going to have his cancer treated. At first, he said he was but he missed his appointments over and over again. His wife had not told me before, maybe because she thought I'd angry? They had decided to put the matter into God's hands. In their home, the curtains were drawn and a few of the children's toys were clustered in the corner. He lay in the bedroom, too weak to walk into the living room. His wife and I talked softly where we stood at the foot of the bed. As she spoke she reached out to caress his feet and toes; an unself-conscious act, a gesture taking for granted his presence, without regard at this moment of his imminent absence.*
3. *The Haitian woman's high pitched labor cries,*
"Jesu, Jesu, Jesu!".
Have passed.
Face moist with sweat, she inspects her son, then she pinches his nose, pokes at his cheeks.
I have seen this before.
To my query, she replies
"We want them to have small noses and dimples."
4. *Ms. Peary smokes cigarettes, one after the other. She doesn't want to see me but her caregiver brings her so she sits on the exam table. I tell her that I would like her to have a CT scan. There is nothing wrong with me she says; I don't need that test. The only thing wrong, she pauses, and in the saddest voice I have ever heard, she told me her heart is broken.*
On account of her husband's death many years before.
5. *Fetal Heart Tones. Pulling up her shirt to listen, it is no longer a surprise to discover the safety pin hidden underneath, Pinned at the waistline of her stretch maternity pants. And also there is the neat bow resting just above her pubic hair, A shiny red cord wrapped about the Mexican girl's round belly, Talismans protecting her unborn.*
A gift for the Future.
6. *My old job. Will I forget H with her face of Africa and her Brooklyn accent? Most days she drank and worried about her daughter. Will I forget the father of L. Who was in and out of prison? I never knew why. His failing heart no longer lub dubbed, just quivered and only briefly.*
Will I forget M with her beautiful smile and diseased breast? Or D with her crooked wig, full of stories and regret?
7. *Use of Force. William Carlos Williams visited that girl with diphtheria (something you have never seen).*
and you had to admire her defiance, her refusal to open her small mouth.
and you had to understand his righteous male doctor rage you'd call it. And then you just had to share his righteous male doctor triumph at overcoming her resistance, at restraining her with the use of force, prying open her small mouth, and saving her life. Though you are not told if her life was saved or whether she forgave his assault.

8. *Once I was with a too-young girl in labor.*
   Who refused to open her legs though the baby was crowning.
   Her fists pulled clumps of hair out of her own scalp like in some Three Stooges episode
   I once saw.
   In my rage I ordered a nurse to each knee to pry open her thighs. In my triumph I caught
   the baby, slick with goo in the nick of time then held that perfect boy.
   For just a moment before turning him over to his crazed-child-mother who by then had
   calmed. Whether she forgave my assault, I never knew.

I wish I could practice Family Medicine again; I feel lost without my work. I hope to complete a book about my patients' lives soon. I have been going to their houses with my cell phone. I record their voices telling their life stories. I had not initially realized how much joy I would feel to hear about their lives. After all, before, I had only been their doctor. Now we are friends.

Post Script

Last night I went to a meeting with some Berkeley students who want to become doctors. They asked about what it was like to be a doctor, and they were earnest and beautiful. Their skin hues ranged from manzanita to ebony to vanilla. They listened when I told them I miss my patients and have loved so many. When I spoke about my patients and how I practice, I felt insecure and worried someone might notice something was not right with me due to my disease.In the end, I felt proud of them and grateful.
When it was over, they asked if they could be in touch with me.
It made me feel happy, so I said yes, please!
In the end, I felt proud of them and glad that they will 1 day have patients of their own.
I told them I appreciated them and the work they will 1 day do for people and for our planet.

Afterword I thought—Screw my disease!
I have work to do.
Thank you, Cynthia Carmichael MD.

Reference

1. Unpublished, Written Collaboratively by the North Richmond Wednesday Morning Breakfast Group (3/5/03).

Chapter 13
Shifting Grounds and Relationships: Some Parting Thoughts

Lucy M. Candib and William L. Miller

We were not unaware, at the time of proposing this book, of the multiple possible interpretations of the title: family doctors saying goodbye to patients, family doctors saying goodbye to their practices and their careers, and family doctors saying goodbye by their departure to the whole concept as they witness the withering of the specialty of family medicine. We asked and coached our authors to address the first two understandings of our use of *Goodbye*. We and our authors are of one mind that real healing takes place within the evolving history between doctor and patient, doctor and family; that the relationship is central to the meaning and importance of the personal connection over the course of decades and generations. As Lynn Carmichael pointed out so many years ago, the word *family* in family medicine refers to the *quality* (what he calls the *process*) of the relationship [1].

Yet over the 2 years of writing, compiling, and editing this book, we can't ignore how the ground under primary care and family medicine has been shifting. We have become increasingly convinced that we are also saying goodbye to that kind of family medicine, which will become increasingly less common, less typical, and less available as the specialization, corporatization, and depersonalization of primary care practice make care within the context of a healing relationship less and less possible. This reality is also true for specialists, who may treasure the long-term care of patients. In primary care, this group includes the pediatricians, primary care internists, women's health clinicians, and mental health professionals, and within the subspecialties in chronic diseases, those clinicians who have maintained relationships with their patients over decades as the disease processes wind down.

L. M. Candib (✉)
Family Medicine and Community Health, University of Massachusetts Chan Medical School, Worcester, MA, USA

W. L. Miller
Family Medicine, Lehigh Valley Health Network, Allentown, PA, USA

© The Author(s), under exclusive license to Springer Nature Switzerland AG 2023
L. M. Candib, W. L. Miller (eds.), *Family Doctors Say Goodbye*, https://doi.org/10.1007/978-3-031-33654-6_13

Already, many of these clinicians are also "bailing out," as the work becomes more regimented, more profit-motivated, and less and less flexible to deliver the dedicated and detailed and time-consuming care within the context of their doctor-patient relationships.

As the ground is shifting, so too is the nature of the relationships that doctors can forge. A person who has known their doctor for decades will wait in the waiting room longer than someone seeing a stranger; the connected patient will forgive the wait because they know that sometimes the doctor took longer with them and other patients had to wait. A random person making an appointment with a doctor unknown to them will have less patience and more reason to seek anonymous care at an urgent care location rather than wait for the individual, who might become their family doctor. Building relationships is much harder now as patients feel less connection to the professional they are seeing, while the clinician feels more pressure to generate numbers, revenue, and income while facing computerized reviews of their productivity and record-keeping.

We also feel compelled to comment on how hard it is for doctors, even family doctors, to acknowledge their emotional selves. The impetus for Lucy to write her chapter with Eydie has to do with this particular challenge: how to face and explicitly address those feelings and hold yourself and the patient together in the process. The years of medical school training in scientific focus and objectivity, linking back to Osler's *Aequanimitas* [2], merge into today's enmeshment with the computer screen. The ability to connect with one's feelings has been squeezed down to an occasional awareness of tears trying to emerge from their tiny ducts. "Not letting it get to you" and "not showing it" are still valued. The spontaneous expression of feelings is equated with weakness in the historically male-dominated world of medicine. Perhaps now, the majority of women in U.S. medical schools will make some dent in this historic standard of conduct, but the forces maintaining it are still very active. The obsession with a narrow understanding of objectivity and rationality continues to quash the richer humanity, the whole person, that includes subjectivity and feeling. How can the importance of relationships with patients and colleagues emerge and be recognized under such a blockade? And how can they come to a shared acknowledgment and mutual acceptance of the sadness of departure and, when relevant, of the growth and healing that have taken place, often for both of them? One of our hopes is that the feminization of family medicine will be a force that strengthens relationship-based care and models more collaborative leadership styles with the gradual supplanting of patriarchal values. For this hope to achieve fruition the profit motive as king must be toppled.

Medical trainees today see where prestige and money are valued, how procedural and one-off episodic care is rewarded, and how time-consuming and unrelenting are the needs of individuals and families who need someone to listen and stay. Some students still look for the emotional and philosophical rewards of continuity, but witness their supervisors and mentors in family medicine being ground down by endless mechanical charting (in so-called medical records that Barry Saver in his chapter calls EBS, electronic billing systems, rather than EMRs) and the moral distress from not being able to do what they know is best for the patients they care deeply about. A study from Norway showed that GPs were more likely to identify their moral distress than other physicians, particularly around services that patients needed and were unable to obtain [3]. Learners are not oblivious to this distress in their teachers. Learners also see the turfing of difficult patients by specialists or hospitalists to any available outpatient doctor and the increasingly unmet needs of the permanent underclasses of the unemployed and underemployed, the poor, immigrant, and refugee individuals and families of color, who because of grindingly persistent structural inequality will never get their needs met by the impersonal one-off medicine of the future. It is all very sad.

Caring clinicians in the private practice of complementary medicine world will pick up part of the slack and bring healing to some seeking relief from pain, but not the care of those without money or those with serious medical problems whose conditions will require care and expensive insurance for hospitalization and testing beyond what the complementary healer can provide. Concierge medicine may work for those ambulatory patients with money but cannot be implemented for those without. Systems will increasingly employ nurse practitioners or physicians' assistants to occupy the roles that family doctors used to fulfill, but they too will get ground down eventually without power and influence in large systems to control the length and frequency of visits and the numbers of new patients assigned. The Medicine of Now is **not** healthcare. It is a business that follows the money. As Don Berwick so recently pointed out, it is all about greed [4]. The people who see healing within the context of relationships have no role to play there because relationships take time and cost money.

What Is the Future?

This could be a depressing way to end a book whose editors and authors believe strongly in the sustaining and healing power of relationships. The eventual realization of equitable universal healthcare coverage, protected from political machinations, would ease some of the challenges but not all. There *is* a future for this kind of relationship, but it may have to be in the realm of the small where it thrives best. The family farm, the corner store, the communities that maintain geographic and social coherence—that's where family medicine can still survive and thrive. People who are looking for that kind of community space are more likely to be able to find or create ways to practice and stay connected. Although rare, we have seen younger family doctors find and build these practices, learning to thrive in briar patches. Direct care practices that also serve vulnerable and under-resourced populations are an example. Likewise, people who want a local, personal, and relational kind of care are more likely to stay in those locations until the small communities can no longer survive ecologically or environmentally. That impending disaster is beyond the scope of this reflection.

Saying goodbye offers a window to all that preceded it. We hope you witnessed, in this book's stories, some of the joy found amidst the work that created the relationships to which the authors said, "Goodbye." All of us loved and cherished this work. We are also encouraged by the enthusiasm of many entering medical students for relational care in the context of local community—until the culture and competitive pressures of medical school constrict their imaginations. In the meantime, we can still guide those learners who continue to long for connection toward a way of practice and a choice of location that might ultimately fulfill their desire to become real family doctors. We encourage the rising generations to risk committing to relationships, to risk challenging the status quo, and to help restore the personal and the wholeness of life. History reminds us that the power of the powerful never lasts. Together, we can hasten that change and continue the work for a more equitable, just, relational, and healthy time ahead. We can hope for that future and cherish the teaching of those learners when we find them, and they find us.

References

1. Carmichael LP. The family in medicine, process or entity? J Fam Pract. 1976;3(5):562–3.
2. Osler W. Aequanimitas: with other addresses to medical students, nurses, and practitioners of medicine. London: H.K. Lewis; 1914.
3. Førde R, Aasland O. Moral distress among Norwegian doctors. J Med Ethics. 2007;34(1):521–5.
4. Berwick DM. Salve lucrum: the existential threat of greed in US health care. JAMA. 2023;329:629–30. https://doi.org/10.1001/jama.2023.0846.

Index

A
Abdominal pain, 93
Academic conferences, 141
Academic medicine, 69, 131, 140
Academic physician, 70
Administrative support, 64
Administrative tasks, 70
Alzheimer disease, 148
American Academy of Family Physicians (AAFP), 142
American economic system, 43
Annals of Family Medicine, 125
Antiretroviral medicine, 150
Anti-war movement, 83
Army scholarship, 36
Automated external defibrillator (AED), 61
Autoethnography, 76

B
Balint groups, 84
Balint principle, 72
Balint, Michael, 74
Bell's palsy, 20
BIPOC, 115
Blood pressure, 152
Brill, Alida, 73

C
Catholic-based hospital system, 115
CDC Prevention Research Center, 132
Chief Executive Officer (CEO), 47
Chronic obstructive pulmonary disease (COPD), 20
Classism, 129
Clinical activity, 104
Clinical care, 64
Clinical interactions, 75
Clinical issues, 94
Clinical license, 65
Clinical life, 65
Clinical relationship, 68–69, 73, 101, 105
Clinical work, 64
Community-based organizations, 142
Community-based residency, 113
Community engagement, 42
Community health center (CHC), 108
Complementary medicine, 157
Computational modeling techniques, 132
Concierge medicine, 157
Constructive criticism, 143
Contract work, 28
Countertransference, 85, 86, 89, 100
COVID-19, 44, 46, 55, 104, 134, 144
Critical life events, 123

D
Dementia, 148, 149
Department of Family Medicine, 63
Depression, 103
Detachment, 137
Diphtheria, 152
Direct care practices, 157
Diversification, 69
Doctor-patient relationship, 69, 85, 90
Doctor's departure, 69
Doctors' emotional responses, 68

Doctors' personal experience, 69
Dysfunctional health care system, 63, 120

E
Education and social work, 2
Educational program, 68
Educational recommendations, 68
Educational setting, 68
8-point program, 137
Electronic billing record, 111
Electronic medical records, 42, 48, 76, 80, 81
Emotional issues, 30
Emotional ownership, 32
Emotions and tasks, 96, 102, 105
Erikson, Erik, 133
Exposure-response prevention (ERP) therapy, 114
External funding, 120

F
Family Health Center of Worcester (FHCW), 112
Family medicine, 1, 2, 27, 29, 56, 73, 84, 120, 141, 143, 153, 155
   engagement, 74
   literature, 70
   and Primary Care, 63
   residency, 148, 149
   residency programs, 24
   resident, 140
   services, 109
   third year clerkship, 40
Family practices, 30
Family therapy, 16, 17
Federal funding, 38
Federally qualified health centers (FQHCs), 39
Fellowship, 67
Feminism, 59
Fetal heart, 152
Financial reward, 67
Financial stability, 68
Financial support, 122
Full scope family medicine, 61, 63

G
General practitioners (GPs), 1, 23, 24
Generalism, 130, 136
Generational tide, 1
Generational wave of family physicians, 2
Geographic and social coherence, 157
Gratefulness, 122
Guilt, 91

H
Health and liability insurance, 27
Health care system, 62, 134
Health center setting, 83
Health insurance, 87
Health system leadership, 41
Hergott, Lawrence, 71
Hospital-based insurance, 25
Hyde Amendment, 115

I
Institute for Integrative Health, 133
Interdisciplinary intellectual ferment, 126
Intergovernmental Personnel Act, 131

J
Jail health services, 110

K
Kaiser protocols, 151
Key skills, 141

L
Leadership, 136
Leadership mentoring, 51
Learning and teaching, 140
Learning new technology, 42
LGBTQI+, 115
Limited Liability Corporations (LLCs), 28
Local mentoring relationships, 56
Long-term clinical relationship, 75
Loxterkamp, David, 71
Lung cancer screening, 151

M
Maikuru Program, 39
Male medicine, 84
Malpractice insurance, 29
Malpractice suits, 29
Medical academia, 70
Medical authority, 84

Index

Medical career, 149, 150
Medical institutions, 68
Medical school faculty members, 121
Medical schools, 30
Medical school training, 156
Medical trainees, 156
Medicine leadership, 41
Mental health issue, 114
Mental health professionals, 155
Multi-generational relationships, 88
Multiple personality disorder, 96
Multiple practice-based research networks, 120
Myasthenia gravis (MG), 20

N
National Cancer Center, 128
National Health Service Corps, 16, 31
Neighborhood Family Practice (NFP), 16, 17, 130
New York State Academy of Family Physicians (NYSAFP), 142
Non-abusive caring clinician, 84
Nurse practitioners, 157

O
Occupational Health, 17
Occupational Medicine, 17
Organ-focused and surgically-oriented specialties, 1
Orthopedic care, 110

P
Palliative care attention, 94
Pandemic, 66
Paramedic, 60
Part-time clinical practice, 111
Part-time transitions, 70
Patient care, 65, 121
Patient diagnoses, 151
Patient-oriented studies, 110
Patient's termination, 74, 100
Pediatric residency, 69
Pediatricians, 155
Personal medicine, 33
Person-Centered Primary Care Measure, 134
Physician "wellness" programs, 31
Physician insurance, 25
Physician retirement, 69

Practice medicine, 31, 81
Pre-matriculation program, 38
Prescription for Health Initiative, 122
Primary care, 110, 155
Primary care internists, 155
Primary health care, 1
Primary medical care, 1, 2
Primary medical care practices, 2
Productivity-based compensation, 116
Professional identities, 88
Program of all-inclusive care for the elderly, 108
Promoting health across boundaries (PHAB), 131
Psychoanalysis, 73, 74
Public health mission, 110

Q
Qualitative research, 75

R
Recognition, 72
Relationship-centered culture, 47
Relationship-centered healing craft, 54
Research career, 113
Research collaborator, 110
Research training, 108
Residency education, 141
Residency program, 115
Retirement, 59, 60, 67, 68, 80

S
Sadness, 91
Scholarships, 36
Second preceptor, 104
Self-compassion, 66
Self-inflicted lacerations, 92
Severe dementia, 108
Sickle cell disease, 149
Social justice-focused missions, 116
Social location, 75
Social security, 28
Society of Teachers of Family Medicine (STFM), 59
Spiegelhalter, David, 126
Spiritual practice, 129, 137
Stories and mental images, collection of, 81–83
Structural racism, 129
Supportive setting, 72

T

Teaching, 104
Termination, 74
Tibetan Himalayan culture, 17
Traditional psychotherapy, 89
Transdisciplinary collaborations, 120
Transference, 85, 86
Truman's checklist, 25

U

Uniformed Services University (USU), 37
U.S. medical schools, 156

V

Vietnam war, 36

W

Wisdom of Practice Initiative, 134
Women's health clinicians, 155
Work first' priority, 63
Workplace transitions, 76, 81

Y

Younger physicians, 68

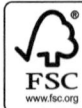

MIX
Papier aus verantwortungsvollen Quellen
Paper from responsible sources
FSC® C105338

If you have any concerns about our products,
you can contact us on
ProductSafety@springernature.com

In case Publisher is established outside the EU,
the EU authorized representative is:
**Springer Nature Customer Service Center GmbH
Europaplatz 3, 69115 Heidelberg, Germany**

Printed by Libri Plureos GmbH
in Hamburg, Germany